CRITICAL A

D0483746

Afraid

"**BERG SERVES UP A FEAST** of facts on four major problems: dysfunctional eating, eating disorders, size prejudice, and overweight. Condemning 'diets,' she instead proposes a wellness paradigm based on the Canadian 'vitality' model, which calls for moderation in eating habits and an active, playful lifestyle. The book contains advice for parents but emphasizes that social change is needed in schools, organized sports, and federal policies that focus too narrowly on antiobesity. Unlike other books on this topic, the unique problems of boys and minority children are also explored. Berg's book is a valuable consciousness raiser. Recommended for public libraries for both parents and concerned professionals."

— *Library Journal*

"*AFRAID TO EAT* **IS A MUST READ** for teachers. The pressures caused by the weight crisis are affecting academic achievement in our youth. It's time for school staff and students to become aware of the size bias pandemic and its consequences, and mobilize to liberate all students to achieve their fullest potential."

— *Linda L. Johnson, MS, Assistant Director School Health*
North Dakota Department of Public Instruction

"**AS THE PARENT** of a daughter who acquired a serious eating disorder in her teens, I can only wish that Frances Berg's book had come along sooner, and health and education professionals had heeded its advice years ago. Thankfully we have it now. Berg provides badly-needed ammunition to those who, like myself, have been groping for weapons in the battle to save kids, both thin and fat, from a lifetime of size oppression . . . Long overdue."

— *William J. Fabrey*
Director, Council on Size & Weight Discrimination

"**AN EXTRAORDINARY** contribution to both professionals and the public. *Afraid to Eat* identifies the cultural, social, physiological, emotional and spiritual issues facing kids today and how these issues collide, resulting in a generation of kids afraid to eat. Ms. Berg is an award winning writer and has a gift for gathering and clearly explaining how these forces influence our children relationally and developmentally.

"A useful chart details dysfunctional eating from inconsistent eating to eating disorders. It is characterized by feeling guilty, ashamed, out of control, fearful of food, frequently uncomfortably full or hungry. *Afraid to Eat* is also a storehouse of charts, graphs, lists, and short articles essential to nutrition professionals working with children and adolescents. Whether you are a workshop leader, counselor, author, educator, coach or in marketing and advertising, these resources will be valuable time after time.

"*Afraid to Eat* demands that as a nation and as health care professionals we deal with these issues in healthier, more effective ways."

— *PULSE*
Dietitians in Sports, Cardiovascular and Wellness

"*AFRAID TO EAT* indicts society for this obsession with thinness and its impact on children's lives, which causes eating disorders, dysfunctional eating, size prejudice and overweight. The obsession and its consequences amount to perpetrating fraud on innocent children. This insightful book shows how to challenge the status quo, and it's easy to read, too."

— *Kentucky Currents, Kentucky Dietetic Association*

"IN HER NEW BOOK, author Frances M. Berg, a national expert in healthy weight education and weight loss fraud, insists that we must allow our children to eat without fear. Regardless of their shape and size, it is time we promote wellness and wholeness in more positive ways for our youth.

"Berg states it is a major health crisis when more than two-thirds of high school girls are dieting, one-half are severely undernourished and one-third are occasionally smoking, mostly in an effort to be thinner. Nearly one-fourth of high school girls are overweight and subject to discrimination, hazardous weight loss attempts and related health risks, and more than one-tenth have potentially fatal eating disorders. One-third feel so badly about themselves and their bodies that they think seriously about committing suicide. Teenage boys mirror these same problems, but to a lesser extent.

"*Afraid to Eat* promotes natural, wholesome eating patterns, healthy food relationships and regular physical activity — a new health paradigm for children. Shifting the emphasis from restrictive ideals, dieting and prejudice, sets the stage early in childhood for normal eating habits, active living and positive self-esteem.

"Teachers will benefit from the discussion of goals for elementary students, advice on how to spot weight problems in athletes and best address body image and self-esteem. If today's children are to grow up with normal eating habits, changes must come in attitudes, lifestyle, society and national health policy."

— *Rochester Times Union, Rochester, N.Y.*

Afraid to Eat

Afraid to Eat

Children and Teens
in Weight Crisis

■

Frances M. Berg

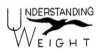
UNDERSTANDING
WEIGHT

Edited by
Kendra Rosencrans

Published by
Healthy Weight Publishing Network

Acknowledgments

It's been my privilege and pleasure to network with many outstanding leaders in the fields of nutrition, eating disorders, obesity, and size acceptance over the years and I thank them for their contributions to this book. I'm especially grateful to Linda Johnson, Karen Petersmarck, Ellyn Satter, Dan Reiff and Joanne Ikeda, and to Kendra Rosencrans for her superb editing, and Ronda Irwin for her dedication and skill in production. Special thanks also to my family, my husband Bert, and children, Kathy, Rick, Cindy and Mike.

Edited by Kendra Rosencrans
Layout and production by Ronda Irwin
Cover photo by
Jon Steinbach, Steinbach Studio
Published by
Healthy Weight Publishing Network
Healthy Weight Journal
402 South 14th Street
Hettinger, ND 58639
Tel:701-567-2646; Fax:701-567-2602
www.HealthyWeightNetwork.com

For the first time in the history of this country, young people are less healthy and less prepared to take their places in society than were their parents.

NATIONAL COMMISSION ON THE
ROLE OF SCHOOL AND COMMUNITY IN
IMPROVING ADOLESCENT HEALTH, 1990

Contents

Foreword

Afraid to Eat is one of the most important books of the decade. This isn't just a book about eating disorders or a book about the problems of children who are overweight. This is a ground-breaking book about an issue in our culture that is affecting almost every single child in ways that range from detrimental to disastrous. Every adult who cares about children needs to understand the message that Frances Berg has clearly articulated here.

The cultural obsession with slimness has reached a level which is seriously hurting millions of our youth. Ms. Berg is one of the few people in the country with a broad enough perspective to piece together the destructive elements which contribute to a previously unrecognized national emergency — an emergency that will get worse unless thoughtful and caring individuals from every quarter take positive action to change the situation.

Children today are flooded with messages telling them that they are unacceptable and unlovable unless they somehow manage to achieve a body size and shape which is biologically sustainable for only a handful of human beings. Whereas natural diversity in other physical characteristics is seen as normal (height, foot size, complexion, nose length), only individuals who fall within the lowest range of weight for height are considered "normal." This message is reinforced in hundreds of ways through the mass media, and it is also unwittingly reinforced by well-meaning adults.

The result is that far too many children see themselves as defective simply because their weight is at a level that is genetically and biologically appropriate for them.

The few children who happen to meet cultural standards for slimness are afraid to gain weight. Even the small weight increases which precede spurts in height in growing children are noted with alarm.

Fear of gaining weight and desperate desires to lose weight are daily realities for many, if not most, of our children.

The restrictions they make in quantity and variety of food are seriously threatening their long-term health, leading to epidemics of disordered eating. What is even more disastrous, however, is the pandemic of self-loathing based solely on body size which compromises the emotional development of the next generation.

Despite the dark picture painted in *Afraid to Eat,* the book is not depressing because Ms. Berg creates a clear vision of what is needed to change the status quo. By integrating the creative thinking of some of the finest minds in North America, she has formulated a set of reasonable, common-sense actions that can turn the situation around.

There will be some people who will consider this book controversial. That is good. We need controversy. We need debate. We need a national awareness of an intolerable situation that will not self-correct.

Afraid to Eat needs to be read, discussed, argued about, and acted upon.

Karen Petersmarck, PhD, MPH, RD
Michigan Department of Community Health
Lansing, Michigan

Introduction

Children and teens today are struggling with a major health crisis that is dominating their lives in often detrimental ways. They live in a culture that tells them their bodies are wrong and promotes destructive values through media, advertising and the entertainment industries. Weight and eating have become an obsessive concern for American children of all ages. These are 21st century youth, the first to reach adulthood in the new millennium. Erosion of their sense of self caused by their weight and eating preoccupation may cripple their ability to meet the challenges of the coming century.

This book outlines a serious and pervasive public health problem, focusing on four major aspects: dysfunctional eating, eating disorders, overweight and size prejudice. It explores the social forces that have shaped these problems, such as cultural expectations and media images, and how they are intimately related. It reviews the growing body of research that documents profound medical and psychological effects of this crisis among children and teens. It looks at the interplay of family, athletics, teen pregnancy, health care and peer pressure on these problems.

Finally, *Afraid to Eat* examines the steps educators, parents, health professionals and society need to take to help young people who struggle with these problems. It will take a paradigm shift to advance the goal of healthy children of all sizes. That change: a unified health approach in which all children receive consistent messages that encourage normal eating, active living, self respect and an appreciation of size diversity.

We must allow our children to eat without fear.

CHAPTER 1

Growing up
afraid to eat

■

America's children are afraid to eat.

It's a fear that consumes, shatters lives, even kills. It's an obsession that dims their joy, their curiosity, their energy and their sense of normal life.

To be overweight is to fail. It's irrational, but kids are succumbing to the same destructive cultural messages about body and weight that plague adults. Instead of growing up with secure and healthy attitudes about their bodies, eating and themselves, many kids fear food and fear being fat.

How can we help them overcome their fears and fulfill their potential as generous, capable, unique individuals?

It's a national public health crisis and we need to take action.

Our daughters and sons are caught — and they need our help. They're not developing the eating habits, lifetime activities and self respect critical to becoming healthy adults with healthy weights.

Some children can't eat normally. Others live with eating disorders. Still others fail to thrive because of the social shame they endure for being large. And we, as parents, educators, health professionals and members of society, have ignored them, punished them, and failed them.

This crisis consists of four major weight and eating problems: dysfunctional eating, eating disorders, overweight and size prejudice. I've been writing and publishing *Healthy Weight Journal*, reporting worldwide research on weight and eating issues, for 12 years. Over that time I've seen an astounding increase in all four problems.

At first I was appalled at the disarray in the health field related to weight and eating problems. Then I was hopeful, believing once the problems were better known they might be solved.

It hasn't happened. Instead, the problems have gotten worse.

I suppose I was naive, believing that once health policy makers understood the problems, they would be willing to make changes. But I underestimated the power of tradition, the marketplace, and the determination of those in power to stay their course.

Yet, these are our children, our daughters and sons, who are growing up afraid to eat. They are desperate to have the "right" bodies, obsessed with the need to be thin, and fearful that they won't be loved unless they reach near perfection. Add that stress to a world already full of drug and alcohol use, violence, sexually transmitted diseases, early pregnancies, and fast-paced media images.

It should come as no surprise in a country where half of adults are dieting that children see, hear and take to heart the cultural ideal that to be thin is to have the best of everything and to be fat is to fail.

These same pressures are growing worldwide, as attested to by our *Healthy Weight Journal* readers around the world, but they are especially acute in the United States and England.

Weight issues have become an obsessive concern for American children of all ages. Clearly it is a national crisis when harmful attempts at dieting are common in the third grade and even earlier. It is a crisis when more than two-thirds of high school girls are dieting and half are undernourished. One in five take diet pills, and many girls as well as boys are using laxatives, diuretics, fasting and vomiting in desperate attempts to slice their bodies as slim as they can.[1]

This is the point to which our weight-obsessed culture has brought us. Our children are the innocent victims.

These are 21st century youth, the first to reach adulthood in the new millennium. How well prepared will they be to meet the challenges of a new century?

The National Commission on the Role of School and Community in Improving Adolescent Health is concerned about this. In 1990, the Commission warned: "For the first time in the history of this country, young people are less healthy and less prepared to take their places in society than were their parents."

A group of girls ages 11 to 17 were asked, "If you had three wishes, what would you wish for?"

The top wish of nearly every girl was to lose weight. Not to cure cancer or save the rainforest or be a millionaire, but to be thin. In another survey young girls said they were more afraid of becoming fat than they were of cancer, nuclear war or losing their parents.[2]

A crisis in eating and weight

Possessed by this fear, many children don't eat normally. They shun certain foods, they diet and they binge. There's a new name for these eating patterns — dysfunctional eating.

First and second graders worry about their weight. Six out of 10 high school girls diet; so do one in four high school boys.

Almost every day, I hear new horror stories about how dysfunctional eating hurts children. Teachers tell me sad stories about the meager lettuce leaves girls put on their plates in the lunch line — and how they droop in class. They tell of the school's star wrestlers, thin-faced and gaunt, who shiver in their winter jackets as they try to focus on writing a test.

Most recently, they tell me about the small girls and boys with fragile, stress-fractured bones, their growth stunted. Some children have been traumatized by radical animal rights groups that come into their schools and deliver graphic propaganda against eating animal-based foods. As a result, these kids won't eat eggs, meat, or milk — the building blocks of healthy growth and development which have for generations made America's youngsters among the tallest, strongest and healthiest in the world. A diet without animal foods must be carefully planned, but these children don't have the skills for this.

I hear from parents that their college-age daughters are eating "zero" fat — if a girl eats ordinary food, she must not swallow it.

College girls who eat normally, or eat meat, may be harassed in their own sororities at Syracuse University in New York, says one of our subscribers, Cynthia DeTota, a registered dietitian who is the campus nutritionist.

Young people who don't eat healthfully set themselves up for nutrient deficiencies and even malnutrition. Teenage girls have the poorest nutrition of any age group in the U.S. For many, chaotic eating, fasting, dieting, bingeing and semi-starvation are disrupting their natural growth.

A recent national study revealed that at the median, girls age 11 to 19 are not getting the nutrition they need for healthy growth and development. The half below the median get less than two-thirds of the Recommended Daily Allowance of iron, calcium, vitamin A and many other essential nutrients, according to the 1995 Nutrition Monitoring report. The lower one-fourth are far below these levels.[3]

Girls who are starving don't think straight. They don't feel well, or act normally.

Girls are also taking up smoking more and more as they grasp at every straw to lose weight. For the first time ever, they now surpass boys in smoking rates. The 1995 Youth Risk Behavior survey shows 20.8 percent of white high school girls are frequent smokers, compared with 18.4 percent of white boys.[4]

One teen in 10 struggles with the most serious kind of abnormal eating — potentially fatal clinical eating disorders. Some are consumed by their eating disorders through college and into adulthood. Others die.

When Christy Heinrich died in 1994 of anorexia nervosa, she was 22 years old and weighed 60 pounds. The Kansas City gymnast had been weight-conscious as long as she'd been competing. But in 1988, a judge at an international competition told the then 16-year-old Heinrich that she needed to watch her weight if she wanted to continue winning.

Her offending weight: 93 pounds.

At the same time, obesity among children and teens has skyrocketed. One in five teenagers is overweight, by the health department's Healthy People 2000 standards, and the rates are much higher among ethnic and racial minorities and the lowest income group. Not only are more youngsters overweight, but they are more severely overweight than ever before. It's a complex problem with no surefire cure. Genetics, inactivity, poor nutrition, and disruption of normal eating habits all play a role.

Meanwhile, large kids struggle with prejudice and stigmatization.

In 1990, a 16-year-old girl wrote to *Parade Magazine* of the anguish and humiliation she had suffered because of her weight and her efforts to reduce.

"I can't speak for all fat people, but I do know that I am not lazy about losing weight. I'm always in the midst of planning a diet, in the middle of a diet or breaking a diet. I've tried sensible diets, liquid diets, crash diets," she wrote. "I've lived my entire life with people reminding me that it isn't okay to be fat. It isn't okay to be 16 years old, 5 feet 6 inches tall, have beautiful hair and eyes, and to be fat. It isn't okay, and it isn't fair."

No public outcry

Body image issues are severe for young people – girls and boys. Yet there is almost no public recognition of these four eating and weight problems and how closely entwined they are.

I'm getting more letters and calls today from youngsters who seem suicidal. A 17-year-old boy from California wrote me a long and anguished letter about the bulimia that is taking over his life: "There is a war going on inside me . . . I don't know what to do. It is tearing apart our family . . . I sometimes feel that death would be better than being fat and having this destroy my family."

Joelyn M., 15, sent me an e-mail message from Pennsylvania, "Can you help me? I'm a vegetarian, but mostly what I eat is lettuce. I think a lot about doing away with myself."

So I was not surprised to see the latest suicide behavior statistics from the 1995 Youth Risk Behavior survey. They show that more than 30 percent of high school girls and 18 percent of high school boys seriously considered suicide during the 12 months preceding the survey, and 21 percent of girls and 14 percent of boys went so far as to make a suicide plan within that year.

These numbers are self-reported and may even underestimate the despair our daughters and sons are feeling. How much does this desire for self-destruction have to do with body image issues, with not measuring up, with sexual violence, harassment, being stigmatized, and depression related to self-starvation?

The shocking part of all these latest reports on nutrient deficiencies, hazardous dieting and suicidal thinking is that there are no headlines, no public outcry, and no public health programs to deal with these problems. There is nothing but public apathy.

The nutrition report I quoted is more than two years old. It never hit the news — and in fact, its own summary hardly mentions the nutrition deficiencies it so clearly documents for teenage girls.

A unifying approach

A new approach is needed to deal with these issues in healthy ways. The goal must be healthy children of all sizes. It must include the intellectual, physical, emotional, social and spiritual development of the whole child, and every child. To achieve this goal, we need to take a unified health approach in which all children receive consistent messages that encourage normal eating, active living, self respect and an appreciation of size diversity. If national health policy experts, health care providers, teachers, families, peers and the media reinforce these messages, the four weight and eating problems will be diminished or prevented.

The health model shown here demonstrates this unified approach based on the principles of good health for all youth at whatever size they are *(figure 1)*. We need to help young people eat normally without fear, build self respect, learn assertiveness and healthy coping skills. We want them to develop their unique potential as lovable, capable, valuable individuals, and take pride in themselves and their bodies at any size, without being stigmatized.

All children deserve this.

Health leaders need to view weight and eating problems within a larger perspective. The big picture is extremely complex, and interrelated. Overweight and its risks cannot be adequately addressed without also considering eating disorders, pressures to be thin, dys-

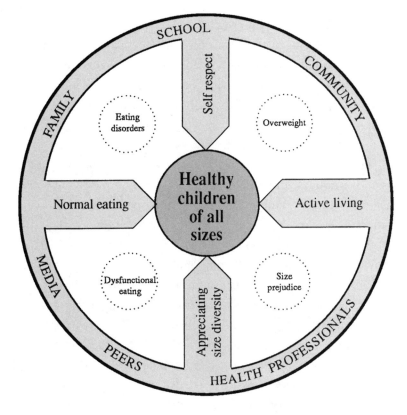

Figure 1

The unified health approach

To achieve the goal of healthy children of all sizes, a unified health approach is needed, whereby all children receive consistent messages which encourage normal eating, active living, self respect and an appreciation of size diversity. If family, teachers, health professionals, peers and the media give these messages to all children, the four major weight and eating problems (dysfunctional eating, eating disorders, overweight and size prejudice) will be diminished.

AFRAID TO EAT 1997

functional eating, size prejudice, body image issues and the failure of weight loss treatment.

How these issues entwine must be considered in developing healthy approaches. Health professionals, educators and parents need to look carefully at all these problems, ever wary of the harm so easily done to vulnerable youth by simplistic solutions.

The old ways of dealing with these problems haven't worked.

The old paradigm holds that all bodies should be at an "ideal" weight and large people must lose weight to be healthy, even though they cannot do this in a healthy and lasting way.

The new paradigm is about wellness and being healthy at every weight. It's about eating in normal, healthy ways, and living actively. It's about self acceptance, self respect and appreciation of diversity in others. Everyone qualifies. Most especially, every child qualifies.

One of the most urgent steps in solving these problems is to empower our half-starved daughters to feed themselves. For many young girls, their current nutrition deficiencies are likely having severe effects on their bones, growth and mental functioning.

Preventive programs based on self-trust will empower children to follow their own body signals and needs. What they most need is help in understanding that they can be healthy and attractive at the weight they are, while growing normally. Along with this they need to feel safe, assured of acceptance, regardless of size, shape or appearance. They need to be liberated from false and narrow images based on appearance, and encouraged to evaluate and combat inappropriate media stereotypes. Programs with this new approach will empower and strengthen all youngsters.

The first step is to stop programs that may be harmful. The next is to encourage healthy, normal eating, while taking steps to prevent the four major problems of overweight, dysfunctional eating, eating disorders and size prejudice, recognizing their interrelatedness. Such a united approach by family, school and health care providers will have positive effects on the dominant culture while strengthening children to withstand the negative messages they are receiving from the culture.

What is healthy for the largest child is also healthy for the thinnest: normal eating, active living, self respect and an appreciation of size diversity.

Canada has already adopted the type of unified approach suggested in this book. Its national program to address weight issues, called *Vitality*, encourages healthy eating, active living and positive self images. Vitality's message is simple: Eat well, be active and feel good about yourself.[5]

Current confusion

The risks of losing perspective by focusing on one or two problems to the detriment of others cannot be overemphasized.

This is the case today, and it's a critical problem. As current U.S. health policy focuses on obesity and weight loss, there is high probability that this is intensifying the problems of dysfunctional eating, dangerous weight loss methods, eating disorders, and the stigmatization of larger youngsters. Following that lead, different groups seek to solve the various problems in often-conflicting ways, and they give out confusing health messages. Most professionals deal with only a few elements of the problems, sometimes working at cross-purposes with others who are equally well-intentioned.

Unlike obesity specialists, who sometimes focus so narrowly on making weight loss happen that they seem unaware of the consequences of their actions, eating disorder specialists are keenly aware of the dangers of promoting weight loss. But they sometimes discount the problems of excessive weight gain.

Few specialists have seemed willing to stand back and view the whole picture. Few have examined the broad tragic network of weight issues that holds so many lives hostage.

We need to do it now.

The crisis continues to grow. The diagram on the next page summarizes the current crisis, and demonstrates how specialists, parents and others work at cross-purposes depending on their area of concern, giving out conflicting messages and allowing the negative aspects of culture to exert a powerful influence on children (*figure 2*).

Health professionals, educators and parents need to look carefully

at the four problems of overweight, dysfunctional eating, eating disorders and size prejudice, aware of the harm that can and is being
done to vulnerable children and teens.

Those who set national health policy, in particular, need to take
a broader view of weight and eating problems since U.S. health
policy sets the agenda for what happens throughout the country. Also
it profoundly influences how the media responds to health issues.

This nation has not dealt well with weight issues. The traditional

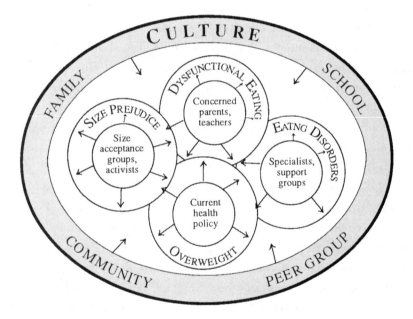

Figure 2

Current weight and eating crisis

Children today are caught in a weight and eating crisis in which national
health policy, health care providers, teachers, parents, peers and the media
give out conflicting messages, working at cross-purposes and allowing the
negative aspects of culture to exert a powerful influence that makes problems
even worse.

view, which is the official health policy view today, is that all large children and adults can and should lose weight.

Health and medical professionals who promote this view assume that any excess weight over a narrow "ideal" is unhealthy, dangerous and expensive to the U.S. health care system; that weight loss is always desirable and healthy for persons over this ideal, no matter how it is accomplished; and that all large persons can successfully lose at least 10 to 15 percent of their weight and maintain it.

They further assume that publicizing the risks of obesity and stressing the importance of thinness is helping people get thin, despite a great deal of evidence to the contrary. And they fear that warning about eating disorders or the risks of weight loss may discourage people from trying to lose weight.

Such fears, along with pressure from the diet industry, have kept eating disorders off of the nation's health agenda in *Healthy People 2000*. This is the document that sets the nation's health goals for each decade. Although several objectives in *Healthy People* deal with trying to reduce obesity before the 21st century begins, none speak to the devastating increase in eating disorders, or the need to stop the harm they do. To me this is shocking and inexcusable.

In this official, traditional view, it is more of a concern that people lose weight than that radical treatment methods are being prescribed for high risk patients, even children, or that underweight and normal weight youngsters are severely restricting their nutrition to lose weight. Or that more and more teenage girls are smoking because of their fear of fat.

Eating disorders, dysfunctional eating and size prejudice are regarded as unimportant, or at least irrelevant to public health's anti-obesity messages. It ignores the possibility that the policy itself might be contributing to these problems.

Many who set national health policy may be influenced by the powerful weight loss industry which pulls in $30 to $50 billion a year in the U.S. alone.

For instance, the nine members of the federally-funded National Task Force on the Prevention and Treatment of Obesity, which is the official authority on obesity treatment and sets U.S. policy, have disclosed for the first time their financial affiliations. This landmark disclosure was required for an article the Task Force published on diet drugs in the *Journal of the American Medical Association (Dec. 18, 1996)*. The list reads like a who's who of the diet industry.

Of the nine members, eight are university-affiliated professors and researchers who have financial ties with from two to eight commercial weight loss firms each. They are consultants, serve on advisory boards, conduct industry research, and receive honorariums and grants from weight loss companies and drug manufacturers of diet pills, most of this support being current or in the previous year.[6]

This disclosure of vested interests illustrates the charges Thomas J. Moore makes in his book, *Lifespan,* that it is "almost impossible to find any boundary between the government, the industry and the medical elite."

He calls it "a closed circle of medical insiders operating without the normal checks and ethical barriers."

Many health officials and researchers do not share the traditional view of emphasizing weight loss, and refuse to support its policies, however, it is the one that currently determines U.S. health policy in regard to weight and eating issues. It is a policy that exaggerates the risks of obesity and minimizes the risks of underweight, malnutrition, dysfunctional eating and eating disorders.

Following are recent examples of this short-sighted bureaucratic policy and its pretense that all is well with obesity treatment.

■ The "healthy weight" table in the 1995 *Dietary Guidelines for Americans* sets a new standard for thinness. It removes the 1990 10- to 15-pound age allowance after age 35, despite strong evidence that a wider weight range is healthy as people grow older, especially for women. All adults with a body mass index of 25 or over, or who have gained 10 pounds since they reached adult height, are told bluntly, "You need to lose weight." The guidelines are published every five years by the U.S. Departments of Agriculture and Health and Human Services.[7,8]

■ "Almost any of the commercial weight loss programs can work," declares a consumer brochure by WIN (Weight-control Information Network) — although it provides no credible evidence for this statement. WIN is a program of the National Institute of Diabetes and Digestive and Kidney Disease. It often seems inappropriately aimed at keeping up consumers' and clinicians' flagging interest in weight loss treatment. The WIN newsletter publicizes the short-term successes of weight loss treatments, and seems to ignore research on weight loss failure. [9]

■ Weight cycling, or yo-yo dieting, was deemed relatively harmless in a special report by the National Task Force on Prevention and Treatment of Obesity. It reached that questionable conclusion by focusing on metabolism, and discounting cardiovascular disease risk and increased mortality. The report urges people not to let their concerns over weight cycling risks deter them from efforts to lose weight. It is promoted and referenced heavily by the diet industry, the Task Force and WIN.[10,11]

■ *Weighing the Options: Criteria for Evaluating Weight-Management Programs,* a 1995 book that reviews available weight loss programs, finds nearly all weight loss methods safe and effective. It also seems to suggest that even more people should undergo stomach reduction surgery. The book defines long-term weight loss as a period of only one year, which might begin on sign-up day and include months of weight loss. However, the American Heart Association says weight loss is not long term unless *maintained* for at least five years, and that virtually all studies show continued regain does not stop after one year. *Weighing the Options* is published by the Institute of Medicine, National Academy of Sciences, a nonprofit group chartered by Congress to advise the federal government on health policy.[12, 13]

Groups like these are pressing hard to launch a major campaign in schools to teach kids the risks of overweight, screen for obesity, get large children on weight loss programs, and persuade insurance companies to pay for it all. I find it hard to believe the primary concern here is for the well-being of large children. Insurance companies, too, often burned by overzealous claims for weight loss programs that didn't work and caused serious injury, are extremely reluctant to back these efforts.

The truth is, we do not have any safe way to effectively treat overweight, even with the new prescription diet pills. Our health and medical specialists should stop pretending that we do.

It's time to confess we don't know the answers. Time to get serious about solving weight problems instead of letting these kinds of leaders, the media, advertising, and the diet industry lead us into deeper trouble.

All this pretense and manipulation of reports and data gets in the way of solving urgent problems. As long as obesity experts and federal health officials insist that their treatments are safe and effective, we are prevented from moving ahead.

Why can't obesity be dealt with in the same way as other health problems, honestly, in a straightforward manner? No one has pretended cancer is cured, then worked secretly backwards to see what went wrong with the cure. We haven't burdened heart patients with the onus of curing themselves. But in the weight field, it happens all the time.

Miracle cures

Over the past 15 years of reviewing worldwide research, reporting, and attending national and international conferences, I've watched a steady stream of miracle cures come and go.

I was there when John Garren introduced his Garren-Edwards stomach balloon to an enthusiastic crowd of admiring physicians. I was there a few years later at a Harvard meeting as he stood alone by his posters, forlorn and rejected, his hastily-granted FDA approval withdrawn.

The attention and enthusiasm had moved on to the promoters of the very low calorie diets, known as VLCDs (800 or less calories), with their "amazing, miracle" results. Large patients lost one-third of their size in months.

I knew Dr. Peter Lindner, one of the great diet doctors of the 1980s, who co-authored with George Blackburn, MD, of Harvard, one of the early studies that seemed to prove VLCD success using safer liquid formulas than those that caused numerous deaths in the

1970s. Theirs became a classic, oft-quoted study that gave much impetus to the liquid VLCD's soaring second wave of "miracles," which again ended disastrously.

Lindner was a magician and cheerleader, urging on his patients and colleagues alike with great enthusiasm. He had many grateful patients, and I feel sure his motivation was to help them. Then why did he grow increasingly despondent? His friend told me it was because, as he confessed before he died, he made a five-year check of his former patients, and not one of them — not one — had kept off for five years any of the weight they lost so successfully for him.

But by then the study had taken on a life of its own. It was referenced, quoted and followed up by hundreds, probably thousands, of nearly identical studies attesting to the success of VLCDs. These are still being presented at scientific conferences and published in scientific journals, even though most hospitals which once embraced them with such enthusiasm have long since quietly dropped the programs.

Liquid diets, even in their failure, were in some places replaced by a very low calorie diet called, oddly, a protein-sparing fast because it contains some real food and supposedly, although this is not true, spares the dieter's muscles. Then came Slim Fast and its imitators filling grocery aisles for a couple of years. Next, thigh cream. Now again, the new prescription diet drugs are all the rage. The latest research shows these drugs don't work very well either, and can be extremely dangerous.

One cult after another, as one scientist complained.

It has been my mission for 12 years to investigate and report the truth about these miracle cures.

And these are just the legal, medically-sanctioned cures. We've reported on more than 200 other fraudulent products: acupressure earrings, appetite patches, hypnosis, body wraps, vacuum pants, battery-operated belts, slimming insoles, herbal teas, Chinese soap, cookies, mushroom tea, starch blockers, cure-all pills, herbals, bee pollen, drinks to detoxify the body. Many have killed. I get heartbreaking calls and letters from victims' families.

And when the victims are children, it's especially hard to bear.

The one method that can work and does no harm is that of moderate eating, living more actively and relieving stress. But it is steadfastly ignored. There's no profit in it.

Current health policy has lost much support among educators and health professionals. For many, it runs counter to their experience in working with weight reduction. They care about their patients, and have seen their best efforts to help fail time and again. They know their patients did not end up the better for it, and they refuse to continue putting more pressure on large people.

Further, several candid reports from some branches of the National Institutes of Health and the National Center for Health Statistics recently have warned that most people who lose weight by any method regain the weight they lose, and that adequate studies of safety and effectiveness are not available for any of these methods.[14]

It's clear that traditional ways of dealing with weight need to be replaced by a paradigm that helps children and does not harm them.

We must allow our children to eat without fear.

CHAPTER 2

Our culture fails
to nurture its youth

■

Modern culture is youth-centered, yet in many ways it does not provide an environment that is nurturing or supportive for the healthy growth and development of our children. In fact, it nurtures serious problems.

This is especially true for girls, which is probably the reason their suicide behavior rates are double those of boys in every category.

"A girl-poisoning culture . . . a girl-destroying place," psychologist Mary Pipher brands our society in her book, *Reviving Ophelia.*[1]

Pipher says that in early adolescence girls are expected to sacrifice the parts of themselves that our culture considers masculine on the altar of social acceptability. They have to shrink their souls down to petite size.

Appearance and, above all, thinness are the criteria by which girls are often judged. Magazines for teenage girls give training in lookism. The emphasis is on makeup, fashion, weight and how to attract boys, with almost no space given to sports, hobbies or careers. In many ways, as in women's magazines, their readers are being sold to advertisers through editorial copy.

What young people want most is to belong, to be accepted. They are always searching, trying out and learning by trial and error. Culture, family, community and friends show them the way. But today family and community are losing out to the stronger influence of pop culture, the entertainment industries and peer group pressure. The messages kids get about how to belong and be accepted are often confusing, conflicting and harmful to their well-being.

Pipher believes that this culture is splitting adolescent girls into true and false selves — one that is authentic and one culturally scripted. They can be authentic and honest, or they can be loved and admired.

Girls fight to preserve their wholeness and authenticity, but most choose to be socially accepted, take up false selves, and abandon their true selves. In public they become who they are supposed to be, she says. Girls struggle with mixed messages, "Be beautiful, but beauty is only skin deep. Be sexy, but not sexual. Be honest, but don't hurt anyone's feelings. Be independent, but nice. Be smart, but not so smart that you threaten boys."

The issues girls struggle with are barely discussed, certainly not in the teen magazines they read or the television shows they watch.

We can help to strengthen girls, encourage emotional toughness and self-protection, support and guide them, but Pipher says the important thing is to change our culture.

"We can work together to build a culture that is less complicated and more nurturing, less violent and sexualized and more growth-producing. Our daughters deserve a society in which all their gifts can be developed and appreciated."

Boys, too, are bewildered by their perceptions of what our culture expects of them. They live in a culture that showcases men as "macho," yet demands equality. It flaunts sexuality, but fears to discuss it. Men are goaded by friends to harass and exploit women and girls. The girls and women they know are obsessed with their bodies, eating and weight, and can talk of little else. Like their sisters, many boys are emerging from childhoods of trauma, violence or sexual abuse.

How thin is thin enough?

Television, movies and other social media probably have the strongest and most dangerous influence on children. At no time in history has the cultural obsession with thinness been more severe. What is it doing to children, particularly girls? Is it sabotaging their chances for healthy weight, healthy self respect and healthy, productive lives?

Studies show that teens today get their values more from the media and friends than from family or community. Both boys and girls are being taught that only thin people are worthy of love, attention and success. They turn that expectation on themselves and their friends, dieting to meet it, hating when they don't.

It seems to me that women on television are thinner this year than last, and that last year they were thinner than the year before. Often now they show us their lean bodies from the side so we can get a good look at how hollow they really are, back to front.

It breaks my heart to see a lineup of thin girls from the side — as with high school basketball cheerleaders, their stomachs caved in, bony clavicles and hip bones protruding. Where are the bodies they have worked so hard to perfect? There's no body. Only bones, arms, legs, hair and that frightening skeletal face, screaming out cheers — or maybe, screaming for help from us adults who have abandoned them.

The cultural lesson: Thin is in, fat is out.

Advertising is a $130 billion industry and the most powerful educational force in America. It has designed the cultural ideals of the late 20th century. "Each era has exacted its own price for beauty, though our era is unique in producing a standard based exclusively on the bare bones of being, which can be disastrous for human health, happiness and productivity," says Roberta Seid, PhD, of the University of Southern California.[2]

Here's how *Newsweek* recently described "the look" of the late 1990s:

"It is a slimmer, more dissipated vision. . . reedy, women with hollow curves and sinewy lines . . . small, frail-looking. . . wan and disengaged . . . austere as the times . . . human coat hangers. . . Clothes fall off them." These images have toppled the "curvaceous supermodels" of the past decade. It's a "return to reality . . . down to earth." The magazine concludes this proves that "men and their appetites" don't rule the world.[3]

Seid writes that in the past, excesses of fashion were severely criticized by social authorities, including doctors, teachers, clergy, parents and feminists. Moralists stressed that there were values more important than outward appearance. But no more. "In the late 20th century all these authorities, especially physicians, seemed to agree that one could never be too thin."

The lookism message is sold thousands of times per day, through television and movies and magazines and billboards and novels and songs. To girls, the command is be thin, avoid fat and you deserve a wonderful life. To boys, it becomes a command to build abdominals, sculpt, become the ultimate muscle man — or you won't be worthy.

And it's a success. Media pressure to be thin is stronger now than at any time in the last 19 years, according to a recent study that compiled statistics for television commercials on diet foods, diet program foods and chemically-based reducing aids, using advertising data from the *Network Television Books*.[4]

The study found diet promotions, nonexistent in 1973, now comprise about 5 percent of TV advertisements. The trend continues to grow, expanding into other media.

Jean Kilbourne, EdD, author of *Still Killing Us Softly: Advertising and the Obsession with Thinness,* argues that advertising overpowers almost every other cultural message through sheer force. The average American sees 1,500 ads per day and spends a year and a half of a lifetime watching TV commercials.[5]

"The tyranny of the ideal image makes almost all of us feel inferior," Kilbourne says. "We are taught to hate our bodies, and thus learn to hate ourselves. This self-hatred takes an enormous toll. . . (in) feelings of inferiority, anxiety, insecurity, and depression."

The ideal body, the ideal myth

The ideal female body type is now at the thinnest 5 percent of a normal weight distribution, say feminist writers. This excludes 95 percent of American women. A statistical deviation has been made to seem the norm, with millions of women believing they are abnormal or "too fat." This mass delusion causes enormous suffering for women and becomes a prison for many, even though it sells a lot of products.

"For women to stay at the official extreme of the weight spectrum requires 95 percent of us to infantilize or rigidify to some degree our mental lives," says Naomi Wolf, author of *The Beauty Myth.*[6]

The increasing pressures to be thin and their reflection in cultural images are vividly illustrated by a 30-year survey of Miss America contestants and *Playboy* magazine centerfold models from 1959 to 1988. These women — cultural icons — have become thinner each year. Now the typical contestant or model weighs in at 13 to 19 percent below expected weight. The clinical criteria for anorexia nervosa is 15 percent below expected weight. To drop weight further is to risk death by starvation, say researchers.[7, 8, 9]

"Pathologically underweight women are being held up as cultural ideals," says David Greenfeld, MD, medical director of the Yale-New Haven Hospital Adolescent and Young Adult Treatment Unit.[10]

Young Olympic gymnasts, the role models of many girls, are becoming younger, smaller and much thinner.[11] The champions are often 16 or younger, weigh less than 90 pounds and are 4 feet, 10 inches or shorter. Body fat may be under 10 percent.

I felt somewhat more hopeful watching the 1996 Olympic games in Atlanta. These gymnasts were older — almost the women athletes we've been hoping for. Then I heard the piping, child-like voice of the injured 17-year-old. Was she almost a woman? I don't think so.

Even children's books reflect and repeat the Western obsession with thinness. One study found that illustrations of young girls have portrayed them as progressively thinner over the past 80 years, while no consistent trend was evident for young boys.[12]

Thin lesson teaches self-hate

"Because our society is so focused on appearance, body image becomes central to our feelings of self-esteem and self-worth, overshadowing qualities and achievements in other aspects of our lives," says Merryl Bear, coordinator of the National Eating Disorder Information Centre in Toronto, Ontario.

"This cultural focus on looking a particular way is taught. Today, being slender has come to have other meanings attached, such as being seen to be in control of one's self and one's life, successful, self-disciplined and attractive."[13]

The media creates a distorted picture of reality in three ways that adversely affect girls and women, says Karin Jasper, PhD, of the Women's Center Toronto.[14]

In portraying women, food and weight issues, the media distorts reality by (1) frequently propagating myths and falsehoods, (2) normalizing or even glamorizing what is abnormal or unhealthy, and (3) creating the false impression that all women are alike by failing to represent whole segments of the real world. These false messages contribute to the prevalence of eating disorders, she says.

Girls and boys believe it, react to it.

Advertising expertly conveys the message to kids that "you're not okay — and here's what you need to buy to fix what's wrong."

High school girls say they are terrified of being overweight. In a study of 326 New York high school girls, 72 percent said they had tried to diet. Currently dieting were 20 percent of underweight, 32 percent of normal weight, and 54 percent of overweight girls.[15]

Leslie Morgan describes how "weight hate" has become a part of the American female identity in an article in *Seventeen* magazine. She calls it an insidious form of self-loathing that is reinforced everywhere a girl goes.[16]

Girls talk about how they look — and how much they hate how they look — on the bus to school, between math and history class, during lunch, after school, when they shop on the weekend. They think about the "cellulite" on their legs, their fat thighs, their not-flat-enough stomach all day long — whether they're on a diet or not, whether they "need" to be on a diet or not. It's an unquestioned part of their life, and it dictates how they feel about themselves and colors how they feel about everything.

Kris Adler of Bala-Cynwyd, Pa., is a 15-year-old girl described as "pretty, smart, very perceptive," happy at home, with lots of friends. She is normal weight, "even slim," but obsessed with perfecting her body.

Adler tells Morgan her story: "Every day at school at least one freshman girl comes up to me and tells me I have a great body. But

2. Our culture fails to nurture its youth

I weigh myself three times a day so the scale doesn't creep up. It should be creeping down. It's not so much that I think I'm fat, it's just that I'd like to take some flesh from one part of my body and put it in other places . . . If I weighed five pounds less I'd be closer to perfect. I'd respect myself more."

Boys are also affected by pressures to shape their bodies to match current perfectionist ideals. They are increasingly being targeted by fitness, muscle and body sculpting magazines and products. Body dissatisfaction is becoming the focus of advertising directed toward males as it has been for females. The value being taught: Only physical perfection is acceptable — you must keep trying.

As boys take in this message, they're responding. Several community studies report an alarmingly high prevalence of severe weight concerns and unhealthy eating habits among male students.

Eating disorder specialists I know tell me they are seeing many more boys with eating disorders today. They blame some of this on the proliferation of muscle magazines telling boys how to get their bodies right.

One study of 321 students, age 12 to 19, found 2.4 percent of the boys along with 15 percent of girls had eating disorder-like symptoms. These boys were at the lower end of the weight range considered normal. They had serious concerns about eating and body shape, even though their concerns were not as serious as those of girls.[17] Boys who don't think they measure up or who are unhappy with their fatness often struggle with dieting and weight loss in much the same way as girls. However, studies suggest that the body concerns of most boys focus on building up lean body mass and sculpting their muscles and "abs," rather than reducing.

This can lead them into extreme forms of exercise and body building. Some specialists see the drive for body shaping as acting out a defense against conflict-laden concerns, often at puberty, related to an overwhelming sense of insecurity, separation fears, boundary uncertainty, and specific sexual identity fears. Emotional issues are expressed as extreme body dissatisfaction and an intense desire to change it.[18]

Still, weight obsession and dieting in young men is far less prevalent than it is in young women — as are eating disorders and the destruction of self-worth.

"How easily weight obsession is dismissed as an inevitable phase of female development," charges Susan Wooley, PhD, professor of psychology at the University of Cincinnati. "Would things be different if our hospitals and clinics were filled with young men whose educations and careers were arrested by the onset of anorexia nervosa, bulimia, or the need to make dieting and body shaping a full-time pursuit?"

We may get the chance to find out.

Body, identity crises

By age 2, girls are watching television and starting their daily exposure to messages that show women who are successful are thin. As preschoolers, they are already hearing that certain types of foods, especially sugar and fat, might make them fat. Of course, they are also seeing and hearing their mothers, teachers, older sisters, and women in general objectify, distrust, and battle their bodies in order to make them acceptably thin.

Six-year-olds understand fat is undesirable, and many know that people who want to lose weight had better diet and exercise. More seriously, a substantial percent of elementary school girls are concerned about their body shapes and have already tried to lose weight. By fourth grade, 40 percent or more of girls "diet" at least occasionally. Those who do not are gathering information and forming values and opinions about body shape and weight management.

Weight preoccupation and body dissatisfaction is occurring earlier and earlier. Forty percent of girls and 25 percent of boys in grades one through five in an Ohio study reported trying to lose weight. About twice as many girls (25 percent) as boys reported restricting or altering their food intake.

In this study, girls who were trying to lose weight seemed more distressed about their shape than nondieting girls, as did dieting boys compared with nondieting boys. Dieting children tended to be heavier, have lower body self-esteem, and greater levels of dissatisfaction with their weight and shape than children with no history of trying to lose weight. However, at this early stage the majority of children did not mention thinness as important to attractiveness.[19]

But in a study of fifth graders, University of South Carolina researchers found more than 40 percent felt too fat or wanted to lose weight, even though 80 percent were not overweight. They found children as young as 9 with severe eating disorders, including anorexia nervosa and bulimia nervosa. The researchers suggest this bodes trouble ahead.[20]

One-third of the girls in a rural Iowa survey of over 400 fourth graders said they "very often worried about being fat" and nearly half of the girls "very often wished they were thinner." About 40 percent of the children dieted "sometimes or very often." Twice as many girls as boys expressed concerns about their size or weight. Some may be laying the foundation for eating disorders. But even dieting and body dissatisfaction falling short of eating disorders warrant concern, warns the Iowa report.[21]

In contrast to restrictive white values, the African American culture seems to define beauty in broader terms. Studies show women of many sizes are acceptable, and black girls don't have to be thin to be thought beautiful. An Arizona study that compared ideals of beauty for 300 adolescent girls found that rigid and fixed images held by white girls contrasts sharply with the more flexible beauty images of African American girls.

Most of the white girls were dissatisfied with their bodies and wanted to lose weight as a way to be popular and "perfect." Over 90 percent were dissatisfied with their weight even when it was normal. Almost as one they described their "perfect girl." She weighed 120 pounds, had very long legs and long blonde hair. Comparing themselves to this ideal, the girls were very dissatisfied with their own weight and appearance. Perversely, these girls did not support their peers who were closest to this ideal, but felt envious and competitive with them. The younger girls in early adolescence were most severely affected by these kinds of self-defeating images.

By comparison, the African American girls in the study held images of beauty which were flexible, fluid and unrelated to a particular size. They were based on each girl's sense of self, style, confidence, and "looking good." Looking good meant a girl was projecting her self-image, establishing a presence, creating and presenting a sense of style, and "making what you have work for you." These girls said they were supported in their efforts to look good by other girls and by family, friends and community.[22]

With attitudes like these, it is no coincidence that black girls in the Youth Risk Behavior survey were dieting at only two-thirds the rate of white and Hispanic girls, or that their suicidal behavior was two-thirds as high.

Famous role models

Mary Evans Young, the English author of *Diet Breaking*, describes what body image issues have meant for four famous women, two British and two American — all role models for adolescent girls. She says their treatment by the media and the public regarding their size, shape and weight, serve to remind all girls and women that their bodies are open to comment, and that any deviation carries the risk of public disapproval.[23]

- *Princess Diana.* Before marriage, Diana is seen in a famous photograph wearing a long, flowing, semitransparent skirt and holding a child. She is "probably a size 12." The public was given no information about her skills or her work but a great deal about her looks and what she wore, reminding others that a woman will be judged on appearance. In the subsequent glare of the media, the press hounded Princess Diana as she lost weight, her hair became blonder, and she grew image-conscious. Once Diana lost too much weight for the media. "There was mock concern" when it was suspected that she might be suffering from anorexia or bulimia. She was criticized for playing with her food and for her faddish eating. "Diana had gone too far . . . she couldn't win. It was a pointed reminder to all of us that our margin of acceptability is very narrow and nonnegotiable, and that failure invites a heavy penalty."

- *Sarah Ferguson.* Before her marriage to Prince Andrew, there is an early impression of Sarah in another photo: "She had just

finished a day's work at a publishing firm and was happily skipping along, smiling at the photographers and film crews . . .
wearing a gathered, calf-length skirt and a navy blue top, probably a size 12 to 14. She looked so ordinary and so happy . . .
a living contradiction of the "thin" edict — she had escaped the
tyranny."

But as Evans Young tells it, the press soon started hounding
Sarah and pulling her apart, criticizing her size and shape, her
hairstyles, her dress sense. Sarah seemed to reel, and there followed a well-publicized series of exercise and reducing scenes.
While the world watched, the new princess turned into a thin and
very different person. But her new, waif-like figure did not ensure a happy marriage. "She has since regained much of that
weight and is again a target for comments about her size and
shape, while Andrew largely escapes hurtful comments about his
size."

- *Elizabeth Taylor.* Over 30 or 40 years, in countless pictures and
  articles the press has chronicled Liz Taylor's relationship with
  food, dieting, fat farms and up and down cycles of weight. "A
  photograph of a 'fallen star' — which means 'fat' — fetches a
  premium price in the press. So long as she is thin, we will all
  want and love her . . . and aspire to be like her. This message is
  not lost on ordinary women. Already feeling a bit insecure, we
  know we need to be loved."

- *Oprah Winfrey.* If ever we needed an example of the way women
  are tyrannized into being thin, Oprah Winfrey is that example,
  says Evans Young. She has lost weight, regained, lost again,
  regained, and shared with the public her experiences, successes
  and failures around food, weight and size. Oprah is a warm,
  caring, compassionate woman who has accomplished much, yet
  she has said her greatest achievement was losing weight.

Evans Young asserts that the treatment dealt famous women like
these "serves to chastise and tyrannize the rest of us." It is a reminder
that women are targets for being sized up in a way that brings other
girls and women into line.

For women, she says, "Our bodies are perceived as public property — up for scrutiny and debate, rather than a personal matter. Because we all have to be very thin, it stands to reason that the fatter ones amongst us will be pressured most. I believe if we accept that even one woman should be oppressed for her body size and shape we are all oppressed by body size and shape — because that is the gauge by which we are all being measured."

Alicia Silverstone, a slim teenage movie star of Batman fame, was ridiculed in the press when she attended the 1996 Academy Awards, because she had gained five or 10 pounds since making her last movie (for which she probably lost weight). Headlines read "Batman and Fatgirl," and "Look out Batman, here comes Buttgirl." She was called "More Babe than Babe."

Silverstone's director was outraged, "What did this child do? Have a couple of pizzas? The news coverage was outrageous, disgusting, judgmental and cruel!"

What message does her experience send to other young women? Will it keep them in line, dieting and starving? Will Silverstone be more careful next time about being seen in public between diets, at what may be her natural size?

Other messages in the mix

When Coca Cola launched a marketing campaign for Diet Sprite, they chose a bony girl listlessly nursing her diet drink and boasted in the advertisement that her nickname was "Skeleton." Public protest forced the company to pull the ad.

"There's something very sick going on here," complained the mother of an anorexic daughter in a Boston consumers group that boycotted Diet Sprite as a result of the ad.

She's right. There is a cultural sickness when emaciated, vulnerable, passive, childlike women are idealized as role models for our daughters.

These advertisements also send other potentially harmful messages to girls. Take the recent Calvin Klein ads that feature thin, vulnerable waifs in sexually provocative poses. Many ads show models as young, wistful and sexually alluring, doing nothing at all but displaying themselves while males reinforce ownership of them by towering over or grasping them, points out Esther Rothblum, PhD, professor of psychology at the University of Vermont.[24]

These cultural messages seem to promote child sexual abuse, which is often linked to eating disorders.

Barbie — one of the most enduring cultural icons for girls — has body proportions that can hardly exist in reality: tiny waist, large breasts, long legs and long, stately neck. She has thighs that never rub together, "big" hair, feet deformed from constantly wearing high heeled shoes, and outfits and accessories that glorify and promote self-absorption, primping, exhibitionism and materialistic behavior.

Young girls want to be like their glamorous dolls, reports a British study that found 9-year-old girls wanted to weigh an average of 11 percent less and were influenced in this by their dolls, as well as by dieting mothers and the thinnest girl in class.[25]

"What better way to ensure a constant supply of these decorative, nonactivist women than to train little girls to emulate this look and attitude at a very early age?" asks Lynn Meletiche, a size-activist, in the *NAAFA Newsletter.* "How better, than by giving them a sample, in the form of a Barbie — and all her attendant accessories, to serve as a constant reminder of the look and attitude they are expected to achieve?"[26]

These attitudes will likely influence the way girls interpret and react to pubertal changes, say Linda Smolak and Michael Levine, professors of psychology at Kenyon College in Gambier, Ohio.[27]

With nearly all the messages about thinness aimed at girls and women, some researchers see strong ties between the American public health crisis over weight and eating disorders and an intentional cultural oppression of women. The attack messages work best when the target is young. And young adolescent girls are most vulnerable.

"I am deeply concerned about what is happening to young girls in our society today," says Paula Levine, PhD, former president of Eating Disorders Awareness and Prevention. "Young girls up until the age of 11 are confident, unafraid of conflict, and willing to say exactly what is on their minds. As they enter puberty, however, they adjust to society's messages about what young women are 'supposed' to be — nice, kind, caring, self-sacrificing, agreeable and compliant."

In classrooms across the country, girls are encouraged to speak quietly, defer to boys, avoid math and science, and to value popularity and appearance over integrity and intelligence.

"If it is true that by the time young girls in this country reach puberty, they are voiceless, their self-esteem is at a low ebb, and they feel anxious, inferior and out of control, is there any more fertile ground for the development of an eating disorder? I think not," says Levine.

She says teenage girls need to recapture the time in their lives when they were confident, courageous, and critical thinkers. "Only when they begin to value themselves as worthy human beings and not as objects of beauty will we begin to win the war on eating disorders."[28]

Setting the stage

But the odds against that are incredibly high.

"'Why are so many girls in therapy in the 1990s?'' asks Pipher. "They are coming of age in a more dangerous, sexualized and media-saturated culture. They face incredible pressure to be beautiful and sophisticated, which in junior high means using chemicals and being sexual. As they navigate a more dangerous world, girls are less protected.''

Yet, this is happening at a time when women have more freedom and independence than ever before. They can command companies, lead hospitals, hold public office and make millions.

Who is pressuring women to be abnormally thin (and men as well, to a lesser extent), and why? And, most critically: How does this pressure affect young girls and children of all sizes? How does it affect girls with eating disorders? What about boys and young men?

Girls have never had more opportunities to develop their minds, yet they grow up feeling as though their bodies are being constantly watched. They learn to feel disconnected from their bodies, as if observing themselves from the outside, especially when they have been sexually abused or harassed, say these experts.

"Girls do not simply live in their bodies but become aware of how their bodies appear in the eyes of boys . . . By seeing their own bodies as images in boys' eyes, they begin to observe rather than to experience their own bodies; their bodies become 'Other' to themselves," say Deborah Tolman, EdD, and Elizabeth Debold, MEd, of Harvard University.[29]

Some are asking: What is "normal" and what is "disordered," for girls growing up in a culture that forces them to live as if their bodies are being "watched, desired and judged?" A culture that encourages girls to use "the power of weakness"; that allows high rates of violence and sexual assault on women, at the same time it demands that the female body be highly attractive and sexual?

Some experts are calling these demands a crime against our children, a monster. "The public conscience is fast asleep," says Naomi Wolf. The public is silent when young women die, she adds.

Is it about women's freedom?

Why is this gaunt stereotype so persistently promoted and the diversity of women being ignored?

From a feminist perspective, the selling of thinness is seen as a manipulative tool to prevent women from gaining power in the work force. For the most part, this travesty is not being perpetuated on women by individual men, who after all have female friends, lovers, wives, sisters, daughters, but by the political power structure and multinational corporations bent on shaping women into the ultimate consumers, perennially dissatisfied with their appearance.

In a searing account, Wolf charges that this power structure unites to force women into a competition of continual striving for thinness and beauty. It's a cruel struggle they can't win.

Through media images and women's magazines, every girl and woman is made to feel a failure in her attempts to perfect her body and face. No matter what her successes in this or other areas of life, she falls short. She feels her body is constantly being judged unfavorably.

As Wolf points out, the adverse effect of self starvation in the ceaseless quest for a thin body is an important factor in keeping women weak, preoccupied, passive, and off track from career ambitions.

Dieting and thinness began to be female preoccupations when women got the right to vote around 1920. Never before had there been idealized "the look of sickness, the look of poverty, and the look of nervous exhaustion." The new, leaner form replaced the more curvaceous one with startling rapidity, Wolf says.

It was a great weight shift that must be understood as one of the major historical developments of the century. It was a direct solution to the threat posed by the women's movement and her newly-won economic and reproductive freedom.

"Prolonged and periodic caloric restriction is a means to take the teeth out of this revolution . . . so that women just reaching for power would become weak, preoccupied, and mentally ill in useful ways and in astonishing proportions," said Wolf.

The cultural fixation on female thinness is not about beauty but female obedience, Wolf charges. It's "about how much social freedom women are going to get away with." Girls are still being admonished to keep their place, to not compete too seriously.

The "good girl" today is a thin girl, one who keeps her appetite for food (and for power, sex and equality) under control, says Kilbourne.

Sexual harassment

Three Canadian researchers think sexual harassment may be one of the important ways in which young girls learn to feel shame, embarrassment, rejection and hatred toward their developing bodies. June Larkin, Carla Rice and Vanessa Russell, Women's Studies specialists at the University of Toronto, organized focus groups in schools in which girls recorded in their journals and shared incidents of sexual harassment.[30]

They suggest that sexual harassment or teasing is a tool of oppression that can alienate girls from their developing bodies and give them a distorted sense of self.

"We have heard countless accounts of this contempt being expressed by their male peers: the girl who is afraid to walk home from school because she is forced to walk past a gang of adolescent boys who routinely call her a 'fat bitch' while they pelt her with stones; the girls who do not want to walk down a certain hallway in their high school because they are afraid of being publicly rated on a scale of one to 10 and coming out on the low end; the girls who are subjected to barking, grunting and mooing calls and labels of 'dogs,' 'cows,' or 'pigs' when they pass by groups of male students; those who are teased about not measuring up to the buxom, bikini-clad girls that drape the pages of various newspapers; and the girls who are grabbed, pinched, groped and fondled as they try to make their way through the school corridors."

Having to ward off comments about being "as flat as the walls," or "a carpenter's dream" created a growing uneasiness about their developing bodies for many of the girls they talked with. A young girl's body image is developed through the messages she receives about her body, her own perception of her body, and her resulting feelings about her body.

As one girl summed it up, "I feel bad about my body and I wish I was a boy."

The Toronto researchers charge that harassing words thrown at girls do not slide harmlessly away as the taunting sounds dissipate. "They are slowly absorbed into the child's identity and developing sense of self, becoming an essential part of whom she sees herself to be. Harassment involves the use of words as weapons to inflict pain and assert power. Harassing words are meant to instill fear, heighten bodily discomfort, and diminish the sense of self."

Sexual harassment is so commonplace it is often perceived as normal, an integral part of female development, and gets largely ignored. Yet it is one of the more pervasive ways that teenage girls are reminded of the hazards of living in a woman's body. Larkin, Rice and Russell see harassment as a pervasive form of violence that contributes to young women's uneasiness about their bodies and results in a disruption of healthy female development.

Sexual harassment may be one of the most important ways in which their "excitement about their developing bodies is crushed," according to these writers. It's a process that brands girls as defective, inferior, and inadequate.

Stigmatizing girls who don't measure up is a way of marking them as different, defining that difference as inferior, and using it to justify oppression. The rejection is experienced by the entire peer group. All absorb the message, and pass it on to younger kids. Stigmatizing large girls not only hurts them, it's also a way to keep thinner girls in line, continuing to focus on diet and weight.

Sexual abuse

Oppression can take many forms.

Harassment, sexual violence, and stigmatization are three interrelated ways that a girl's resources are weighed down, leading to eating and body struggles, say Larkin, Rice and Russell.

Sexual violence is the most graphic and oppressive tool for subordinating women, they suggest. Often girls report they use bingeing and purging as a way of expelling the frightening feelings that come from being sexually traumatized. They may develop eating and weight struggles, cut or burn themselves, or dissociate from their bodies as a way of disconnecting from the source of their vulnerability. Rape, incest or sexual abuse in childhood is reported by 30 to 40 percent of women, but is much higher in eating disordered patients, they report.

Until very recently, sexual abuse was discounted as a factor in eating disorders, in much the same way it was disavowed by Sigmund Freud in the 19th century in his treatment of "hysterical" women who told him they were victims of incest and sexual abuse. The field of eating disorders was dominated until nearly the 1990s by patriarchal specialists who refused to take childhood sexual abuse seriously. Now it is accepted as a known risk.

It's about shame

The consequence of this abuse is shame, often felt as the result of humiliation and failure to measure up to high standards of appearance. Shame is the response to being violated, harassed and stigmatized, the overwhelming sense of being inadequate and wrong. Shame as a result of harassment and oppression can make girls want to disappear, become invisible, disconnect from their bodies while engaging in "relentless body criticism and improvement in an effort to bolster their shattered self-esteem," say the Toronto specialists.

Rice says this can make girls vulnerable to chronic dieting and eating disorders, "For someone faced with unrelenting discrimination in the form of blatant public hostility and disgust, demeaning and dehumanizing jokes, and unwanted advice . . . losing weight becomes an attractive means of attempting to retrieve lost self-esteem as well as gaining and achieving success."

Girls who stop eating when boys call them "cows" or "pigs" may actually be taking understandable steps toward gaining approval by creating a more acceptable body, rather than behaving in pathological ways, as was formerly believed, explain feminists.

Girls shut down

As girls move into adolescence, their growing preoccupation with their bodies has been interpreted as expressing the need for male approval. But feminist writers suggest their motivation may be more about struggling for some power and self-protection.

The Toronto writers say ogling by males quickly teaches girls the risks inherent in their maturing bodies. They find leering can be a process used by males to select those females who will be the target of their future sexual and abusive comments and behavior.

They quote Marian Botsford Fraser, "At some point in their physical development, all female children lose the protection of baby fat and barrettes and become prey in a game in which there are rules only if the laws are broken . . . The worst messages come from men. I have watched the way that grown men feel free to look at young girls . . . lets his eyes slide all over the body of a pretty teenage girl walking by . . . grunts when he encounters two teenagers young enough to be his daughters . . . mutters, 'check out the hot blonde' to his buddy; the hot blonde is not yet 16."

Some girls attempt to take control of their bodies by shrinking them until the self seems to disappear.

Prevention of eating disorders and dysfunctional eating needs to begin by dealing with the sexual harassment of young girls as their bodies begin developing.

"I think if the women's movement has failed young girls in this country, which it clearly has, then they need a girls' movement," Levine says.[31]

Women must speak out forcefully about the dangers of the obsession with thinness, says Kilbourne. "This is not a trivial issue; it cuts to the very heart of women's energy, power and self-esteem. This is a major public health problem, one that endangers the lives of young girls and women."

CHAPTER 3

Dysfunctional eating
disrupts normal life

■

We are seeing big changes in the way kids eat today, changes in what they eat, and how they eat.

You may recognize the eating patterns. The fourth grader who eats only a small amount of each food on her plate, never feeling really satisfied, because she's afraid of getting fat. The 12-year-old who comes home to an empty house and eats continuously on whatever snack foods are available. The junior high girl who skips breakfast and lunch, has a candy bar and Diet Coke after school, finds a way to skip the evening meal with her family — and then goes on an eating binge in the evening. The wrestler who fasts for two days before his match to make weight, then eats nonstop for the next day or two. The high school student who refuses meat, eggs, milk or any foods she imagines might make her fat.

Dysfunctional eating is a new term to describe the kinds of inappropriate, abnormal, or disordered eating behaviors which disrupt normal life, but not to the level of clinical eating disorders.

This kind of eating hasn't been investigated in much detail. Yet, concerned leaders have been writing about various aspects of it for more than a decade.

Dieting — a form of dysfunctional eating — starts in children as young as age 7 or 8, and by age 11 is so common that some research-ers are calling it the norm for girls in America today. Children are growing up with skewed attitudes toward food, eating and weight because of fear of fat. They are turning away from normal eating and mealtimes with family to a restricted, restrained and chaotic form of eating.

A growing number of studies document this disturbing trend. More than half of 14-year-old girls in a study of 1,000 suburban Chicago girls had already been on at least one weight loss diet.[1] Similarly, 30 to 46 percent of 9-year-old girls and 46 to 81 percent of 10-year-old girls in a California study had disordered eating, re-stricting their food due to fear of fat.[2]

If abnormal or dysfunctional eating is so prevalent, why don't we know more about it? What are its effects? How can it be measured?

It's time to take a closer look.

What is dysfunctional eating?

Dysfunctional eating is eating that is separated or disjoined from its normal function and normal internal controls.

In contrast to normal eating, dysfunctional eating most often serves other purposes than nourishment, such as to shape the body, seek comfort or pleasure, to numb pain, or to relieve stress, anxiety, anger, loneliness or boredom. It is regulated by inappropriate external and internal controls — "will power," a planned diet, counting calories or fat grams, or emotional or sensory cues (seeing or smelling food).

Though often the reason for eating is to relieve stress, it does not do this well. Instead of relieving pain, dysfunctional eating often makes the situation worse. It is common to feel guilty, ashamed, uncomfortably full, to regret or berate oneself for having eating or, if unsatisfied, to feel ravenously hungry and fear triggering a binge. There may be a sense of loss of control.

Dysfunctional eating exists on a continuum between normal eat-ing and eating disorders, and may be of mild, moderate or severe intensity *(see charts on pages 54-55)*. Individuals may move back and forth across the continuum, returning to normal eating after bouts of dieting, or restricting so severely they go on to develop debilitating eating disorders from which they cannot recover alone.

Dysfunctional eating includes the various kinds of disturbed eating patterns which have been called restrained, disordered, disconnected or emotional eating, as well as chronic dieting syndrome. It can also mean consistently eating too much and overriding natural satiety signals.

In contrast, normal eating is controlled by an internal system that regulates the balance of food intake with expenditure, through hunger, appetite and satiety signals, so that a person usually eats when hungry and stops when full and satisfied. Normal eating is flexible and includes eating for pleasure and social reasons. In normal eating a person follows regular habits, typically eating three meals a day and snacks to satisfy hunger. Normal eating nourishes the body for health, energy and strength, enhancing feelings of well-being.

This is the way babies, small children and even animals feed. They eat when they're hungry and stop when full. But even before puberty many American girls no longer eat this way.

Studies suggest that dysfunctional eating is extremely prevalent, especially among girls and women. It appears to be increasing and striking at younger ages as the cultural drive for thinness continues to intensify. And it is widespread. As many as 50 to 80 percent of girls and women in the U.S., age 11 and up, say they're trying to lose weight. Increasingly, they are joined by teenage boys and men who are responding to new advertising pressures to reshape their bodies.

Dysfunctional eating is unlikely for infants, small children and others who don't diet or overeat, or have not learned to interfere with the normal eating process.

Dysfunctional eating includes three general patterns: 1) chaotic or irregular eating; 2) consistent undereating; and 3) consistent overeating of much more than the body wants or needs.

■ **Chaotic or irregular eating.** Many young people eat in chaotic or irregular ways: fasting, dieting, skipping meals, snacking, restricting their eating at times and bingeing at others. They may have a fear of fat, body dissatisfaction, and a strong desire to change their bodies in ways they perceive as more socially desirable. This pattern may also include people who eat erratically be-

Dysfunctional eating: a description

Contrasted and compared with normal eating and eating disorders

	Normal eating	Dysfunctional eating *mild moderate severe*		Eating disorders
Eating pattern	Regular eating habits. Typical pattern is to eat three meals and snacks to satisfy hunger.	Irregular, chaotic eating — often overeat or undereat, skip meals, fast, binge, diet. Or usual pattern is of overeating or undereating much more or much less than body wants or needs.		Patterns typical of anorexia nervosa, bulimia nervosa, binge eating disorder, other eating disorders.
Function, purpose of eating	Eat for nourishment, health, energy. Also pleasure and social reasons. Eating enhances feelings of well-being, makes one "feel good."	Eating often for reasons other than nourishment: to shape body, seek comfort or pleasure, numb pain, relieve stress, anxiety, anger, loneliness or boredom. May feel uncomfortable after eating, or have feelings of remorse, guilt, shame.		Eating almost entirely for purposes other than nourishment or energy, as for body shaping, to numb pain, relieve stress.
Use of hunger, appetite and satiety to regulate eating	Eating regulated by internal signals of hunger, appetite and satiety. Eat when hungry, stop when full and satisfied; usually hungry at mealtime.	Eating often separated from normal controls of hunger, appetite and satiety. May be regulated by "will power," a planned diet, calories or fat grams, emotional or sensory cues, such as sight or smell of food.		Eating regulated predominantly by external and internal controls other than hunger and satiety.
Prevalence	Infants, small children, those who don't diet or override body signals. At this time, probably higher rates among males.	Chaotic eating and undereating affect many girls and women in U.S.: as many as 50 to 80% age 11 and over report trying to lose weight. Increasing numbers of boys and men. Consistent overeating may occur for both males and females.		Estimated prevalence is 10% of high school and college students, 90-95% of them female.

Afraid to Eat: Children and Teens in Weight Crisis. Copyright 1997 by Frances M. Berg. All rights reserved. Published by Healthy Weight Publishing Network, 402 South 14th Street, Hettinger, ND 58639 (701-567-2646; Fax 701-567-2602).

Dysfunctional eating: effects and relationships

	Normal eating	Dysfunctional eating *mild*　　*moderate*　　*severe*	Eating disorders
Physical	Promotes health, energy, strength, and the healthy growth and development of youth.	May typically feel tired, apathetic, lacking in energy, chilled, risk of stunted growth with undernutrition. Decreased bone development, higher risk of bone demineralization, fractures. Delayed puberty, decrease in sexual interest.	Physical effects may be severe. Mortality reportedly as high as 18% for anorexia nervosa and bulimia nervosa.
	WEIGHT: Normal weight for the individual, expressing genetic and environmental factors. Any weight within wide range, usually stable.	WEIGHT: Any weight within wide range depending on genetic potential. Eating pattern may cause weight to decrease, cycle up and down, remain stable, or increase.	WEIGHT: Any weight within wide range, depending on genetic potential and the disorder and its expression.
Mental focus	Promotes clear thinking, ability to concentrate.	Risk of decreased mental alertness and ability to concentrate, narrowing of interests, loss of ambition, turning inward.	Diminished capacity to think, memory loss, extreme narrowing of interests.
	FOOD THOUGHTS: low key, usually at mealtime. For women, 10-15% of time awake may be spent thinking of food, hunger, weight.	FOOD THOUGHTS: Increased preoccupation with food. Thoughts often focused on eating, weight, planning when and what to eat, counting calories or fat grams. Thoughts of food, hunger, weight may occupy 20-65% of time.	FOOD THOUGHTS: Focused most of time on food, hunger, weight. For untreated anorexia about 90-110% of time awake (extra 10% includes dreaming), bulimia 70-90%.
Emotional	Promotes mood stability.	Potentially greater mood instability — highs and lows. May be easily upset, irritable, anxious, have lowered self-esteem. Increasingly concerned and preoccupied with body image. Increased risk of eating disorders.	Greater risk of mood instability and functional depression.
Social	Social integration; promotes healthy relationships with family, peers, community.	Less social integration, more risk of feeling isolated, self-absorbed and self-focused, stigmatized, disconnected from society, lonely. May have less interest in values of generosity, sharing, volunteering; less sense of community.	Social withdrawal, isolated from family and friends, avoidance of and by peers, alienation, often eating alone, worsening family relations.

cause of illness or insufficient food.

- **Undereating.** Many girls and young women, and some males, eat less food than meets their daily needs and requirements for healthy growth and development. They may be "dieting successes," and may develop anorexic eating patterns, even though they do not meet the clinical criteria for anorexia nervosa. Today these are frequent reports: teenage girls with daily intakes consisting of only lettuce, or an apple or bagel, or perhaps "half a raisin"; a college sorority in which members pay a penalty if they eat any fat at all; a dancing troupe in which fat may be eaten but not swallowed. They are able to successfully restrict their eating so that they maintain a thin body and weight which is lower than normal, given their genetic and environmental heritage. Also, undereating may occur because of depression, alcoholism, or other factors.

- **Overeating.** Many children and adults may eat more food on a daily basis than their bodies want or need, eating past satiety, and well above maintenance and growth needs. Body size is not to be taken as an indicator of this type of dysfunctional eating; it cannot be assumed that large persons eat abnormally, or past the point of satiety. Some individuals overeat from emotional or stress-related reasons, such as to gain comfort, deal with anger, or relieve anxiety or boredom. Others overeat from habit. Still others may simply eat more because an abundance of good tasting food is readily available. Disruptions of hunger, appetite and satiety regulation, such as in Prader-Willi syndrome, may also fit in this category.

Physical effects

The person with dysfunctional eating behaviors may often feel tired and lacking in energy, especially when undernourished. Children risk stunted growth and intellectual development, according to poverty studies worldwide. Bones may not develop normally. Or bone demineralization may begin, leading to stress fractures. Puberty may be delayed and normal sexual development arrested.

Dysfunctional eating affects weight, yet in its various forms it is associated with a wide range of weights as genetic potential interacts with environmental lifestyle factors. Associated with chaotic eating, dieting, and bingeing, weight will often cycle up and down in "yo-yo" fashion. Consistent undereating can be expected to result in a stable weight lower than normal for that person. Overeating will probably result in higher weight than might be normal for that individual, likely increasing year by year.

Mental focus

One of the most dramatic effects of dysfunctional eating related to undernutrition is its impact on personality and the thought process. It can have severe emotional effects. The undernourished girl with dysfunctional eating easily becomes moody and upset, is irritable, anxious, apathetic, increasingly self-absorbed, and focused on her appearance. As interest in food takes over she may retreat from social activities and lose interest in school work, career, family and friends. She may feel lonely, alienated, disconnected from society. She tends to lose interest in the values of generosity, sharing and caring, and pull back from volunteer activities and helping others.

This may be the girl primarily occupied with a boyfriend who wants to marry right out of high school. Anorectic girls tend to be popular with boys, explains psychologist Mary Pipher — they are slim, very feminine, passive and eager to please.

The increase in food preoccupation that comes with hunger is clear in the wartime Minnesota Human Starvation study, and more recently has been researched by Dan Reiff, MPH, RD, and Kim Lampson Reiff, PhD, a husband-wife eating disorder team in Mercer Island, Wash.[3]

In their book, *Eating Disorders: Nutrition Therapy in the Recovery Process,* the Reiffs use a food preoccupation scale. Patients are asked to write total conscious time spent thinking about food, weight and hunger at three periods in their lives (currently, at its highest, and at its lowest) and to give their age and weight at each. This includes time spent in shopping, preparing food, eating, thinking about eating, food cravings, purging, weighing, reading diet books, suppressing feelings of hunger, using strategies such as smoking or chewing gum to distract from hunger, and thinking about or discussing weight.

The Reiffs have tested more than 500 eating disordered patients on this scale. Untreated anorexia nervosa patients spend 90 to 110 percent of waking time thinking about food, weight and hunger (the extra 10 percent includes dreaming of food, or having sleep disturbed by hunger). Bulimic patients report about 70 to 90 percent.

With dysfunctional eating, they suggest these thoughts may occupy 20 to 65 percent of waking hours. Women with normal eating

---

Eating Attitudes Test (EAT)

Sample questions

Choose the answer that best applies:
Always - Very often - Often - Sometimes - Rarely - Never

1. I am scared about being overweight.

2. I stay away from eating when I am hungry.

3. I think about food a lot of the time.

4. I have gone on eating binges where I feel that I might not be able to stop.

5. I cut my food into small pieces.

6. I am aware of the calorie content in foods I eat.

7. I feel guilty after eating.

8. I vomit after I have eaten.

9. I think about burning up calories when I exercise.

10. I stay away from foods with sugar [or fat] in them.

11. I feel that others pressure me to eat.

12. I like my stomach to be empty.[2]

FROM GARNER AND GARFINKEL'S EATING ATTITUDES TEST
CHILDREN'S VERSION, BY MALONEY, ET. AL./AFRAID TO EAT 1997

habits, who are buying and preparing food for the family, will probably spend about 10 to 15 percent of waking time thinking about food, weight and hunger, says Dan Reiff.

In these studies, the intensity of food preoccupation is directly related to how much weight is lost and the degree and duration of semi-starvation.

In the Minnesota Starvation study, 32 male volunteers cut their daily food intake in half (to about 1,570 calories) for six months and lost one-fourth of their weight. The formerly idealistic, good-humored men became argumentive, sarcastic, self-centered and preoccupied with food. They spent much time collecting recipes, studying cookbooks and menus, planning how to deal with mealtime food, and toying with and dawdling over their food. Food was their central topic of conversation — the men talked of little else but hunger, food and their weight loss.[4]

Eating disorder risk

Many health professionals and others are concerned that the current high prevalence of dysfunctional eating will lead to increased rates of eating disorders. This is a controversial issue, yet it is clear that many girls and young women who begin dieting and restricting food do go on to develop eating disorders.

A recent review in the *Renfrew Perspective*, an eating disorder newsletter, reported that several one- to two-year longitudinal studies have shown up to 35 percent of normal dieters advance to pathological dieting. Of pathological dieters, 20 to 25 percent progress to partial or full syndrome disorders. From 15 to 45 percent of those with partial syndrome progress to full syndrome eating disorders within one to four years.[5]

How dysfunctional eating starts is not well understood. The effects of one bout of dieting may perpetuate more disturbed eating, say Linda Smolak and Michael Levine, eating disorder specialists. Abnormal eating patterns may begin through following the example or encouragement of parents or friends. When children begin dieting early, they may gradually develop more intense and disrupted eating patterns that lead to fully-developed eating disorders.

"Such disregulated eating may take the form of more stringent and frequent dieting, as well as binge eating. Thus, the children who are already dieting during elementary school may be at risk for developing eating disorders because of the physiological and psychological effects of caloric restriction and weight loss failures."

Another pathway may be cultural pressures to be thin.

"Girls who put enough stake in the importance of thinness may find it necessary to go to extremes in order to attain the desired look, resulting in body dissatisfaction, dieting and exercising for weight control and, perhaps, eating disorders," say Smolak and Levine. Their research shows a subgroup of girls in grades one to five already believes "thinness is important in determining whether a girl is pretty."[6]

Dysfunctional eating may not be so very different from clinical eating disorders. For some it's just a matter of degree. It is no longer possible to dismiss patients with severe eating disorders as uniquely pathological, as was often done in the past. They may be expressing what many other girls and women across the eating spectrum are feeling.[7]

Chronic dieters and those who fear fat experience the same kinds of mental and physical harm as eating disordered patients, to the degree that they practice self-starvation, abuse of diet pills, purging and similar behaviors.

Survival traits

Can some of the abnormal effects of disturbed or dysfunctional eating be explained as survival traits that kept our ancestors alive through periods of semi-starvation?

I believe they can. Prehistoric humans must have frequently feasted for weeks on carcasses of mammoths or beached whales, followed by a famine that may have lasted as long as the proverbial seven lean years. During famine their bodies would have shut down to conserve fuel, not just with slowed heart rate and metabolism, but in every activity. Growth stopped or was severely stunted. Fat consumed would have been routed to storage, filling empty fat cells where possible, instead of being used normally. Sexual activity and fertility shut down; it was more critical to care for the young than to procreate.

Ultimately, as starvation advanced, even children and the elderly would be abandoned, as Colin Turnbull shows us so vividly in *The Mountain People,* his report of an east African tribe of Ik hunters driven from their homes into a stark barren land. The starving Ik people came to fear and distrust each other, and seldom spoke. Cruelty took the place of love as their culture broke down. They lost religion, rituals, spirituality, all sense of moral obligation. Men and women went out alone to forage for food, returning empty-handed to avoid sharing with crying children, weakened parents or spouses.[8]

Today, U.N. relief teams working with starving people see this same sad desertion of family to save oneself.

At the same time, starvation causes high stress. There is no peace for starving people. They crave food and focus on this one overriding need. A useful survival trait, this kept our starving ancestors from giving up — lying listless in the cave awaiting death — and instead drove them out to hunt food, in spite of danger, howling blizzard or physical exhaustion. When food was again plentiful, people feasted. They binged, and ate voraciously. And their bodies' natural efficiency may have increased to guard against the next famine.

Without this internal regulation, matching energy outgo to input, adjusting for fat loss, the human race could hardly have survived. But it's an ancient legacy that haunts today's dieter. She eats less — but then craves food and burns fewer calories. And her body rebounds quickly from weight loss.

Cultural pressures encourage dysfunction

American culture today encourages dysfunctional, disturbed and disruptive eating patterns. Youngsters are being coaxed to overeat and at the same time, told to restrict eating. They are being persuaded to override their internal control systems of hunger and satiety, and take on the responsibility of reshaping their bodies according to the narrow ideals proscribed by society.

Normal eating is not being encouraged. Instead, it's easy to eat too much, to ignore the satiety signals that say we've eaten enough.

We have an abundance of cheap, good-tasting foods, easily available. A culture of eating for pleasure or recreation has developed, shaped by billions in advertising dollars.

Studies show overeating is being encouraged. People are eating out more, and they favor fast food chains and restaurants where they think they get more for their money.

Advertisements for Pringles Right Crisps show people eating 10 or 20 chips at a time. Ritz Air Crisp ads implore kids to "inhale them." And Baked Lays Potato Chips challenges, "Betcha can't eat just one — bag."

Restaurants are offering larger servings, larger meals, more abundant buffets with many food choices. A recent study in *Restaurants USA* found customers expected larger quantities of food in 1993 than in 1991, and that people think of large servings as getting better value for their money when they eat out.[9]

A subscriber in London recently sent me a newspaper clipping titled "Portions out of all proportion" that decried America's "elephantine cuisine." The writer compares the size of foods: hot dogs (350 calories in the U.S., 150 in Britain), cookies (493 vs 65), ice cream cone (625 vs 160), muffin (705 vs 158), nachos (1,650 vs 569), and a meal of steak and fries (2,060 vs 730). Until recently, our large muffins were called "jumbo muffins," the article notes, now they are simply "muffins."

The Cheesecake Factory heaps food "practically a foot high on its plates and proudly serves up a 12-ounce burger. As for the cheesecake, each slice has about 700 calories. It claims it tried to serve lower-calorie slices but nobody wanted them," the article said.

And I detect a bit of a British sniff which, yes, we probably deserve: "Europeans are a lot more quality conscious . . . Americans just want value for their money, and base value on size."

Ironically, at the same time that we are being persuaded to overeat, dieting and thinness are even more heavily promoted. Thinness is a potent advertising theme being used to create body dissatisfaction and sell products from diet pills to fashions, from perfume to cigarettes. The health community has joined with advertisers and the media in urging both children and adults to slim down their bodies in so-called "healthier" ways.

Both extremes promote dysfunctional eating — eating for purposes other than to nourish the body for optimal health and performance. They ignore the fact that our bodies are wonderfully designed to maintain balance through internal regulating systems.

Moreover, there is an intense fear of food in the U.S. today. People are confused and worried about the foods they eat. It's no wonder, with the contradictory scare messages in the media.

"I've never known so many people to be so worried about what they eat, or so many who think of the dinner table as a trap that's killing them," laments Julia Child, the noted chef and author. Child is involved in the "Resetting the American Table" project which enlists nutritionists, chefs, educators and product developers in trying to help people rediscover the joys of eating while moving toward healthier food choices. It promotes eating good food with friends and family as a pleasurable and healthful experience.

The project confronts the damaging effects of "our largely single-focused messages, especially messages urging restriction of food choices or based on fear of disease."[10]

Family attitudes

Family attitudes about weight can set the stage for developing disturbed eating. These attitudes may be evident in frequent family dieting, using restriction, compulsive eating, overeating or excessive exercising to control anxiety, disparaging comments, and obsession with appearance, say the Reiffs.

They point out that a father or mother who disrespects or disapproves of the body shape or weight of the other parent teaches a child to fear such responses from her parents, boyfriends or spouse. Parents and siblings who criticize overweight people may convince the child that she must never become overweight or she too will be unacceptable.

The uneasy relationships that mothers have with food and their bodies are mirrored in their daughters at very young ages. Ellyn Satter, RD, an eating disorder specialist and international specialist on childhood feeding, advises parents to model normal eating. "If you diet constantly . . . If your eating is fragile and chaotic and fraught with anxiety, (your child's) chances are increased of learning to eat in much the same way."[11]

Satter says parents should purchase, prepare and serve the food, but then allow the child to choose what and how much he or she will eat. Unfortunately this natural division of responsibility is often violated by parents with rigid or restricting eating styles, who try to take over their children's eating, she reports. This sets the stage for disruptive eating styles. "But even the fat child is entitled to regulate the amount of food he eats," Satter says, even though that might be difficult for parents to accept.

Making food a battleground can contribute to eating problems for children. In a nondiet program led by Christie Keating of Victoria, British Columbia, teenagers shared the following family eating experiences, as quoted in the HUGS Club News.[12]

"My mom knows I hate mushrooms and I told her I would throw up and she made me eat it and I threw up."

"If we eat too much, we get this story about being greedy."

"My mom won't give me any more, even if I'm hungry."

"My grandmother serves me, so I can't pick."

"Cooked peas and carrots make me gag and my parents wouldn't let me eat anything else until I was finished."

"If you breathe through your mouth, you don't taste it."

"We used to stuff our mouths with the foods we didn't like and then ask to go to the bathroom."

"If I eat all my dinner, then I can have dessert."

Disruption of normal eating may occur when parents fear a child is gaining too much weight and begin to restrict food. Such deprivation diets can foster disordered eating and weight gain, warns Laurel Mellin, RD, MA, University of California, San Francisco. She reports that obese youngsters are at greater risk for developing disordered eating than normal-weight youth.[13]

Never put a child on a diet, Satter advises. "Diets are not an option. Restricting food intake, even in indirect ways, profoundly distorts developmental needs of children and adolescents."

She says it's time to define problems of childhood obesity in ways they can be solved, rather than continuing to set patients up for failure by putting them on weight loss diets. "In my view, no person

has the right to impose starvation on another, even if that other person is your child. Withholding food profoundly interferes with a child's autonomy, and you will both pay the price."

Research needed

The adverse factors associated with dysfunctional eating and its high prevalence make further study imperative. Indeed, it is amazing how powerful the associations reveal themselves when we see the big picture. Much research is needed in these areas.

How can we identify and measure the patterns of dysfunctional eating? If it is unhealthy, how can it be prevented? What are the causes of related emotional changes: too few calories, nutrient deficiencies, weight loss or depleted fat cells? How can children and parents rediscover normal eating?

Normal eating itself needs study. What is it and how can it be measured?

In focusing on the effects of dysfunctional eating, I do not mean to suggest that nutrition is the major factor in good mental and physical health, but rather, that each person has a baseline of adequate nutrition, and when this is disrupted it causes severe disruption of normal life and a diminishing of mind, body and spirit. Only when the food supply is stable can people eat and live normally, as we interpret this today. With adequate nutrition and regular eating habits, they can focus on developing their full potential through a wide range of work and interests. They can afford the luxury of being generous, sharing, caring, and reaching out to others.

Research basis

The concepts of dysfunctional eating I've brought together are defined here for the first time, yet they are based on the insight and research of numerous leaders in the fields of obesity, eating disorders and size acceptance. Much of it is contained in our 1995 special report, *Health Risks of Weight Loss. (See also Appendix D for references discussing this concept.)*

Still most striking to me are the classic Toronto milkshake studies of the early 1980s showing that the more milkshakes restrained eaters

consumed before dinner, the more food they ate. And I've been moved by the wartime Minnesota studies of men who opposed war but went on an austere six-month diet to help starving people in war-torn countries. Even more distressing are Turnbull's terrible revelations in *The Mountain People* of what really happens to society and family life during starvation. More recently, I've been alarmed to learn how much of their lives many dysfunctional eaters devote to thinking about their hunger and their weight, and how little to concern about others.

And I'm reminded that everywhere in our country, today and every day, women and young girls are doing this to themselves and having it done to them by health professionals, advertisers and con artists, as they're pressured to become thinner and ever thinner.

In the 12 years I've been publishing *Healthy Weight Journal,* I've read nearly every scrap of research and insight on this topic (my library on weight and eating research has been called the most extensive in the world, and I believe it may be).

What I'm seeing is an increase in dysfunctional eating, its engulfing of ever younger children, and national increases in related adverse effects, while many in the health and medical communities (with their shepherds, the diet companies) continue to increase pressure on Americans to lose weight.

Changing all this cannot be easy. But perhaps bringing together what is known about disturbed eating, and placing it into a framework as in the dysfunctional eating charts will help. If women and men understand how severely dieting disrupts their lives, will they be so quick to discard life's richness for the preoccupation of watching a few pounds come and go?

Perhaps they will awaken with a start, restore normal eating in their homes, reach out with love and caring, and become — with their children — whole again in mind, body and spirit.

This is my hope.

CHAPTER 4

Eating disorders
shatter young lives

■

As American adults continue to obsess about weight and diet, it is hardly surprising that eating disorders among their children have risen to crisis levels.

While overweight may carry health risks over a lifetime, some eating disorders, like anorexia nervosa, can be deadly and take but a few years to kill.

Several estimates suggest the severity of these disorders. One textbook estimates that 10 to 15 percent of anorexia nervosa patients die of their illness.[1] Dan Reiff and Kathleen Kim Lampson Reiff report that follow-up studies they reviewed show death rates as high as 18 percent for anorexia and bulimia.[2] And the Canadian National Eating Disorder Information Centre in Toronto warns that both anorexia and bulimia can have severe physical and emotional effects, and in 10 to 20 percent of cases can be fatal.[3]

Eating disorder survivors find the road to recovery difficult. For some there are irreversible physical and mental changes due to malnutrition and purging. While in the grip of the disorder, health, jobs, school and relationships all suffer — and rebuilding can be a nearly insurmountable challenge. Less than half of patients, about 44 percent, recover well, according to these sources. About 31 percent are intermediate, and 25 percent have poor outcome.

Eating disorders steal time and concentration from other relationships and growing-up activities. They can be associated with alcohol and/or drug abuse, which may increase medical and mental complications. Sufferers lose energy, irritate easily, are lonely and driven to keep their disorder a secret.

Common symptoms include fatigue, lethargy, weakness, impaired concentration, nonfocal abdominal pain, dizziness, faintness, sore muscles, chills, cold sweats, frequent sore throats, diarrhea and constipation, according to Allan Kaplan and Paul Garfinkel in *Medical Issues and the Eating Disorders.*[4]

"I have many regrets. I lost a number of friends, hurt a lot of people I care about," laments one young woman who recovered from anorexia nervosa and bulimia nervosa. "My memories of the last 16 years are spotty and dim. In fact, there have been many major events, such as my sister's wedding, that I have no recollection of. Eighty to 90 percent of my time was spent in (eating) behaviors. My behaviors overtook my life and I essentially lost 16 years of living — years that I can't have back."[5]

The father of a child with an eating disorder said, "She has withdrawn into her own world. She's lonely and is missing out on all the fun and exciting things during her teenage years . . . I have cried many times over this."[6]

Families of eating disordered youth are in a difficult situation. They see their child behaving in destructive ways and feel helpless and frustrated. They may try to gain control over what and how much the teenager chooses to eat. Some police washrooms and search through drawers for diet pills or laxatives. Moms and dads struggle both with the child's problem eating and their own concerns over injury to growth and development. The eating disorder may take over and dominate family life.

Many specialists in the field are convinced that the current high rates of eating disorders in the U.S. are the inevitable result of 60 to 80 million adults dieting, losing weight, rebounding, and learning to be chronic dieters. The majority of chronic dieters are women.[7]

Prevalence

Prevalence has been difficult to determine because of the extremes sufferers take to hide their disorder, limitations of assessments, and public health apathy in compiling national statistics. Current figures are probably under reported. I feel sure we would have more accurate statistics by now if eating disorders had not been kept off the nation's Healthy People 2000 agenda, in what I regard as an effort to protect vested interests in the weight loss industry.

⌐About one in 10 teenagers and college students suffer from eating disorders, 90 to 95 percent of them female, according to the National Eating Disorders Organization. Michael Levine recently compiled figures for the February Eating Disorder Awareness Week giving a "conservative estimate" that 5 to 10 percent of post puberty females are affected by eating disorders which cause significant misery and disruption in their lives.[8] The Canadian Centre reports somewhat higher figures: in addition to those North American women who have anorexia and bulimia, another 10 to 20 percent engage in some of the symptoms on an occasional basis.

These are not solid statistics based on national figures, but rather smaller studies, and many experts suggest the figures are actually much higher.

Although not conclusive, there is much evidence that eating disorders have increased over the past 30 years, according to Harold Goldstein of the National Institute of Mental Health. The Institute suggests that cases of anorexia and bulimia have doubled over the past decade. Sharp increases have been found among females age 15 to 24, and a study in Scotland found the incidence of anorexia increased over six times between 1965 and 1991.

Most of the eating disorder specialists I network with and many writers in the field are saying that the prevalence has increased in the past decade, eating disorders are striking at younger and younger ages, and they are affecting many more boys and young men.

Nancy King, MS, RD, co-author of *Moving Away from Diets* and a registered dietitian who works with disordered eating in southern California, says she now sees 7- and 8-year-old children with nearly full-blown eating disorders. "Many pediatricians are not recognizing

Eating disorders

■ Anorexia nervosa

Patients with anorexia nervosa refuse to maintain weight at what is minimally normal for age and height (they weigh less than 85 percent of expected weight), and have an intense fear of weight gain or becoming fat. They have disturbance in body image, causing undue influence on self-esteem, and amenorrhea if female, defined as the absence of at least three consecutive menstrual cycles.

Two types are:

- **Restricting type**: severely restricts food without regularly binge eating or purging.

- **Binge eating/purging type:** severely restricts food and binges or purges (vomiting, laxatives, diuretics, enemas).

■ Bulimia nervosa

In bulimia nervosa the individual has recurrent episodes of binge eating. An episode includes eating, in a discrete period of time, an amount of food larger than most people would eat, and a sense of lack of control over what or how much one is eating during the episode. It includes recurrent inappropriate compensatory behavior to prevent weight gain, such as induced vomiting, misuse of laxatives, diuretics, enemas or other medications, fasting or excessive exercise. Both binge eating and the compensatory behavior occur on average at least twice a week for three months. Self-evaluation is unduly influenced by body shape and weight. (The disturbance does not occur exclusively during episodes of anorexia nervosa.)

Two types are:

- **Purging type:** uses regular purging behavior (induced vomiting, misuse of laxatives, diuretics, enemas).

- **Nonpurging type:** uses other inappropriate compensatory behaviors, such as fasting or excessive exercise, but does not regularly engage in purging.

■ Eating disorder not otherwise specified

The largest category is *Eating disorder not otherwise specified*. Individuals in this category do not meet the definitions for either anorexia nervosa or bulimia nervosa.

Examples are:

- All criteria met for anorexia nervosa except amenorrhea.
- All criteria met for anorexia nervosa except, despite weight loss, current weight is in normal range.
- All criteria met for bulimia nervosa except frequency of binges is less than twice a week or for a duration of less than three months.
- An individual of normal body weight who regularly engages in inappropriate compensatory behavior (such as induced vomiting) after eating small amounts of food.
- Repeatedly chewing and spitting out large amounts of food, without swallowing.
- Binge eating disorder.

• Binge eating disorder

A subtype under the category *Eating disorder not otherwise specified,* binge eating disorder is defined as having recurrent episodes of binge eating, which includes eating in a discrete period of time an amount of food larger than most people would eat, and a sense of lack of control over eating it. The individual has marked distress regarding binge eating, and engages in binge eating on average at least two days a week for six months. (The binge eating is not associated with regular use of inappropriate compensatory behaviors and does not occur exclusively during the course of anorexia nervosa or bulimia nervosa.)

At least three of the following must be part of the binge episode:

- Eating much more rapidly than normal.
- Eating until uncomfortably full.
- Eating large amounts of food when not hungry.
- Eating alone because of embarrassment about how much is eaten.
- Feeling disgusted with oneself, depressed, or very guilty about eating.[1]

*Source: Diagnostic criteria for eating disorders. Diagnostic and Statistical Manual, Fourth Edition, 1994. American Psychiatric Association, Washington, DC/*AFRAID TO EAT 1997

it's an eating problem when a child this young loses 12 pounds over the summer. They're not yet in puberty!"

About 9,000 people are hospitalized annually in the U.S. for the treatment of eating disorders, according to Robin Sesan, PhD, director of the Brandywine Psychotherapy Center Wilmington, Del.[9]

Widely regarded as a modern problem, eating disorders have been known for centuries. Earlier it was thought eating disorders are most prevalent in middle and upper socioeconomic levels, but there is increasing recognition that they affect people of all income levels, genders and ethnic groups.[10]

Eating disorders usually consist of two sets of disturbances: first, are the problems related to food and weight, and second, problems concerning relationships with oneself and others. They are extremely complex, arising out of both emotional problems and eating disturbances, within a culture that puts great emphasis on thinness and appearance. Some problems may be rooted in families that are overly controlling or disengaged, or who have problems they are unable to acknowledge or deal with openly. Puberty is a critical time.

Often sexual abuse or trauma will be an initiating event. Some specialists see eating disorders as survival strategies developed in response to harassment, racism, homophobia, abuse of power, poverty, or emotional, physical or sexual abuse.

Dieting disorders

The term "eating disorder" is somewhat misleading because it implies the problem is learning to eat normally again. Given the complex behavioral and psychological components of eating disorders, it isn't that simple.

"Eating disorders should be called dieting disorders, because it is the dieting process and not eating that causes the initiation of both anorexia nervosa and bulimia nervosa," says Joe McVoy, PhD, an eating disorder specialist in Radford, Va.

McVoy says the term "eating disorder" seems to indicate something is wrong with the eating process, whereas what happens is a conscious choice to restrict one's food intake or diet, which leads to starvation and ultimately the disorder.

"Onset of an eating disorder typically follows a period of restrictive dieting; however, only a minority of people who diet develop eating disorders," says the American Dietetic Association in its position paper on eating disorders.[11]

There is debate over whether dieting can lead to eating disorders. Experts linked to the weight loss industry, who often promote dieting, do not want to believe this happens.

Yet, dieting is increasingly being regarded as an important risk factor. A study of 15-year-old girls in London linked dieting to the development of eating disorders. Those initially dieting were significantly more likely than nondieters to develop an eating disorder within one year. Only 21 percent of the girls were dieting at the beginning of the study, but they were eight times more likely to develop an eating disorder later.[12]

The ADA warns against promoting weight loss to persons with binge eating disorder or other eating disorders. When youngsters come for help with weight loss, the ADA position paper on eating disorders recommends counseling on body image issues and how to stop the pursuit of thinness. It may be healthier, the paper says, to suggest that young people accept themselves at or near their present weight, stop binge eating and learn how to prevent future weight gain.

Anorexia nervosa

"When I first started to eat strangely, all I would eat were sweets, and that wasn't any good. Then I got into just eating salads, just lettuce and diet pop, and that wasn't any good. Then I got into pretty much not eating at all, and that wasn't any good," said a former anorexic patient quoted in *Eating Disorders*.[13]

In Levine's statistics, anorexia nervosa affects about one to four of every 400 girls. The Canadian Centre estimates it affects 1 to 3 percent of women in the population.

Anorexia has had some high-profile victims. Singer Karen Carpenter. Gymnast Christy Heinrich.

Actress Tracey Gold, of the ABC sitcom "Growing Pains," was only 12 when her pediatrician first diagnosed her anorexia. Four months of psychotherapy seemed to get the problem under control and she gained weight, up to 133 pounds by the time she turned 19 in 1988. It was too much, she thought. To lose weight her endocrinologist put her on a 500-calorie-a-day diet and in two months she had dropped to her goal of 113. But during the next three years her weight kept dropping, until in January 1992 at 80 pounds she was hospitalized and had to fight to save her life. Two years later, "now rosy-skinned" and feeling "healthy enough to know I don't want to lose any more," she still panicked at the thought of reaching 100 pounds, and kept her weight at 92 pounds.[14]

Female athletes and dancers are at high risk for anorexia nervosa. As many as 13 to 22 percent of young women in selected groups of elite runners and dancers have the disorder. Two studies of female dancers cited by Jacqueline Berning and Suzanne Steen, authors of *Sports Nutrition for the 90's,* found between 5 and 22 percent had anorexia nervosa, with a higher incidence among young women competing in national versus regional performances.[15]

In anorexia nervosa, by definition, the individual is more than 15 percent under expected weight, fears gaining weight, is preoccupied with food, has abnormal eating habits, and has amenorrhea, or if male, a decrease in sexual drive or interest. There are two types: one simply restricts food; the other restricts food and either purges regularly, or binges and purges both, according to the *APA Diagnostic and Statistical Manual.*[16]

Changes occur in behavior, perception, thinking, mood and social interaction. A sense of heightened control and control over food seems important to the person with anorexia. Pleasure and enjoyment during eating are replaced by guilt, anxiety and ambivalence. Mood tends to be depressed, irritable, anxious and unstable often leading to increased social isolation. Compulsive exercise may be a part of the disorder.

Symptoms are usually evident: emaciated appearance, dry skin, sometimes yellowish, fine body hair, brittle hair and nails, body temperature below 96.6, pulse rate usually below 60 beats per minute, subnormal blood pressure, and sometimes edema, say Kaplan and Garfinkel.

Initially, these are similar to symptoms associated with a restrictive diet: light-headedness, apathy, irritability, and decrease in energy. Then the consequences of prolonged semi-starvation begin to set in and effects worsen. Duration of the disorder may range from a single episode to a lifelong illness.

Hospitalization may be required depending on body weight, the amount and rapidity of weight lost, severe metabolic disturbances, certain cardiac dysfunctions, syncope, psychomotor retardation, severe depression or suicide risk, severe bingeing and purging (with risk of aspiration), psychosis, family crisis, inability to perform activities of daily living, or lack of response to outpatient treatment programs. Most severely underweight patients, under 20 percent below average weight for height, and those who are psychologically unstable will require a residential health care setting.[17]

Families as well as patients usually need psychotherapy.

In explaining what it is like to be a male with an eating disorder, Michael Krasnow writes in *My Life as a Male Anorexic* that he began to feel fat as early as age 11, but it was as a high school freshman that "fat feelings" began to take over. He dropped swiftly from his normal weight of about 135 pounds. Now 27, he maintains 75 pounds on his 5-foot-9 frame.

"When I first got this anorexia, I tried to get better, but now I just don't care," says Krasnow. He does not get together with friends, "I haven't had a friend in 10, 15 years."

He refuses to drink water and says he fears if he let go of any of the rules he makes for himself, he would lose control. "It would all fall apart. If I took one cup of water a day, I'd be drinking two gallons a day. Pretty soon I'd be a compulsive eater — that's what goes through my mind — I won't be able to stop."[18]

Bulimia Nervosa

"I can't stop throwing up. I try, I really do. Yesterday, I promised myself I wouldn't do it anymore. I tried to keep myself busy. I cleaned house, played with the cat, prayed . . . But I don't want to gain weight. I can't do that! I never want to be fat again. I'll never go back there. Nothing is worse than that pain . . . My joints even hurt. I feel so old. My hair looks horrible; and it keeps falling out. I find it all over the place. My mouth is so full of sores, it's gross! I can't even walk around the house standing straight any more. I'm in a daze. I can't focus. But I can't stop. I feel so trapped. Please help me . . ." said a patient from Lemon Grove, Calif., as quoted in *The Healthy Weigh*.[19]

Bulimia nervosa affects 1 to 3 percent of middle and high school girls, 1 to 4 percent of college women, and 1 to 2 percent among community samples, according to figures compiled by Michael Levine. A recent study of college freshmen found 4.5 percent of females and 0.4 percent of males had a history of bulimia nervosa, say the Reiffs. The National Eating Disorder Information Centre in Canada reports 3 to 5 percent of women in North America have bulimia.

By definition, a person with bulimia nervosa goes on an eating binge at least twice a week, eating a very large amount of food within a discrete period and then tries to compensate either by purging or nonpurging behavior. As the disorder progresses it develops into a complex lifestyle that is increasingly isolating, with depressed mood and low self-esteem.

Vomiting is the most common form of purging, which includes taking laxatives and diuretics. Some bulimics binge and purge many times a day. Patients with bulimia may be of normal weight and seem physically healthy — except for the tell-tale signs of vomiting behavior: finger calluses or lesions on the dominant hand from stimulating the gag reflex (especially in early stages when stimulation is needed to induce vomiting), "chipmunk" cheeks from stimulation of the salivary glands, erosion of enamel especially on the surface of the upper teeth next to the tongue.[20]

The consequences of self-abusive purging behavior become increasingly obvious as the frequency and duration increase, and include hair loss, fatigue, insomnia, muscle weakness, edema, dizziness, sore throat, stomach pain or cramping, bloating, bad breath and bloodshot eyes. Cardiac arrhythmias affect 20 percent and require emergency treatment. Ipecac syrup abuse may lead to death through cardiomyopathy, myocarditis.

Up to one-third of anorexic individuals develop bulimia nervosa. Bulimia was only recognized in 1980 and listed by the American

Psychiatric Association in its *Diagnostic and Statistical Manual.* In 1987 this was replaced by the term bulimia nervosa. It is unclear whether the disorder has been a hidden syndrome, or is relatively new.

Bizarre behaviors

Many of the physical and mental abnormalities of eating disorders are known to chronic dieters and people who severely restrict their food intake.

The bizarre eating behaviors common to anorexia nervosa are also typical of those described under other starvation conditions. In Ancel Keys' well-known Minnesota Starvation study of the effects of famine in male volunteers who reduced their food intake by 50 percent and lost 25 percent of their weight, the men exhibited many similar behaviors.

As they lost weight, their food interest intensified. The men talked food, fantasized about food, collected recipes, studied cookbooks and menus, and developed odd eating rituals. They would dawdle up to two hours over a meal, toying with their food, cutting it in small pieces, adding spices, sometimes in distasteful ways, trying to make it seem like more and of more variety. They were possessive about food, hoarded food, and spent much time planning, preparing and eating food saved from meals. They ate their allotted food to the last crumb, and some licked their plates. They grew angry when they saw others wasting food.[21]

Feelings related to this kind of behavior are explained by a woman who had recovered from anorexia nervosa and bulimia nervosa, in *Eating Disorders.*

"While anorexic, my body not only anticipated eating, it reveled in it. Being starved and hungry makes the experience of eating more intense — almost sensual. The feeling is analogous to what is experienced when drinking water when extremely thirsty, sleeping after being totally exhausted, or urinating after one's bladder has become overly full. What is usually somewhat ordinary becomes exciting — something to look forward to in an otherwise painful and lonely world. This made changing behaviors so that I no longer experienced intense hunger extremely difficult.''[22]

Yet restoring full nutrition brings dramatic improvement to both the mind and body for sufferers of anorexia nervosa, as it did for Keys' volunteers.

Other eating disorders

Some eating disorders don't fit neatly into these diagnostic criteria. They may have many features of anorexia or bulimia, but involve different eating behaviors, such as repeatedly chewing and spitting out, but not swallowing, large amounts of food.

Levine calls these *atypical eating disorders,* and finds prevalence rates of 2 to 13 percent of middle and high school girls, and 3 to 6 percent of post puberty females in the community.

Binge eating disorder is included in this group. This newly-identified disorder meets the criteria for bulimia nervosa except that individuals do not regularly engage in purging behavior and do not meet the criteria for being unduly concerned with weight and shape. They eat large amounts of food at least twice a week, in a relatively short time, with a sense of loss of control. They may be of average weight, but most often are overweight.

This disorder was first described in 1959, and is similar to what has been called "compulsive eating." Research on binge eating is still in its infancy.

Excessive exercise

One of the fastest growing eating disorder behaviors in the past five years is excessive exercise or exercise addiction to lose weight or sculpt the body, says McVoy. Many anorectic and bulimic patients deal with some form of exercise dependency, explains Karin Kratina, MA, RD, an exercise physiologist and registered dietitian at the Renfrew Center in Florida.[23]

Excessive exercise aimed at weight loss is regarded as a secondary dependency, usually to an eating disorder, says Kratina. Physical activity takes priority over everything else for the exercise-dependent individual. He or she follows stereotyped patterns, continues exercising even when it causes or aggravates a serious physical disorder.

There may be severe withdrawal symptoms upon stopping exercise.

"Stress injuries are common, and frequently the person exercises right through an injury so it can't heal properly," reports Kratina.

Anorexia and bodybuilding have many similarities, points out David Schlundt, PhD, an eating disorder specialist at Vanderbilt University in Nashville. "There are special diets, use of diuretics, steroid use, obsessive exercise, very low fat diets, and so on. An obsession with changing size and shape of the body leads to extreme and sometimes dangerous changes in diet, exercise and substance abuse."[24]

One of the reasons eating disorders are increasing among young men is likely a result of this new obsession with muscles and body sculpting. Boys are reflecting a dissatisfaction with their natural bodies and an intense desire to alter their appearance, McVoy says.

Links to sexual abuse, violence

Childhood abuse violates the boundaries of the self, and increases the risk for eating disorders. Violence, physical or psychological abuse, trauma and sexual abuse are invasions that can have extremely harmful effects.

Sexual abuse is a common experience of many eating disorder patients, says Susan Wooley, PhD, professor of psychology and co-director of the Eating Disorders Clinic at the University of Cincinnati Medical College.[25]

Until very recently, the importance of a history of sexual or physical abuse was minimized by the mostly male therapists who dominated the field in research, publishing and conferences. Wooley calls it the "concealed debate" which women therapists held in conference hallways, and is finally being recognized.

The National Women's Study, a national random sample of 4,008 adult women in the U.S. who were interviewed at least three times over the course of one year, found that women with bulimia nervosa were twice as likely to have been raped (27 percent vs 13 percent) or sexually molested (22 vs 12 percent), and four times as likely to have experienced aggravated assault (27 vs 8 percent) as women without an eating disorder.

Eating Disorder Warning Signs

Anorexia nervosa

- Significant or extreme weight loss (at least 15 percent with no known medical illness)
- Reduces food intake
- Develops ritualistic eating habits such as:
    a. Cutting up meat into extremely small bites
    b. Chewing every bite a large number of times
- Denies hunger
- Becomes more critical and less tolerant of others
- Exercises excessively (hyperactive)
- When eating, chooses low to no fat and low calorie foods
- Says he/she is too fat, even when this is not true
- Has highly self-controlled behavior
- Does not reveal feelings

Bulimia nervosa

- Makes excuses to go to the restroom after meals
- Has mood swings
- May buy large amounts of food and then suddenly it disappears
- Unusual swelling around the jaw
- Weight may be within normal range
- Frequently eats large amounts of food (a binge), often high in calories, and does not seem to gain weight
- May decide to purchase large quantities of food and eat it on the spur of the moment
- Laxative or diuretic wrappers found frequently in the trash can
- Unexplained disappearance of food in the home or resi-

dence hall setting

Binge eating disorder

- Frequently eats a large amount of food that is larger than most people would eat during a similar amount of time
- Eats rapidly
- Eats to point that is uncomfortably full
- Often eats alone
- Shows irritation and disgust with self after overeating
- Does not use methods to purge

Additional signs of related eating disorders

- Makes excuses to skip meals and does not eat with others
- Develops a tendency to be perfect in almost everything
- Conversation is mostly focused on foods or around body shape
- Often hears other people's problems but does not share her own
- Is highly self-critical
- Worries about what others think
- Thinks about weight and body shape most of the day
- Begins to isolate more from friends and family
- The odor of vomit is in the bathroom regularly
- Repeatedly chews and spits out food — does not swallow large amounts of food
- May purge and yet not binge eat[2]

NOTE: The more warning signs a person has, the higher the probability that the person has or is developing an eating disorder.

NATIONAL EATING DISORDERS ORGANIZATION 1994/AFRAID TO EAT 1997

Over half the women with bulimia reported a lifetime history of some type of criminal victimization event compared to less than one-third of women who did not have an eating disorder (54 vs 31 percent).

Twelve percent of women with bulimia nervosa had been raped as children, at age 11 or younger, compared with 5 percent of women without an eating disorder. The age at the time of rape predated the age of the first binge episode in all cases, suggesting childhood sexual abuse as a causal factor.[26]

Even so, the true extent of sexual abuse is unknown due to silencing of the victims and their reluctance to disclose abuse even to therapists trained to help them in this area. Wooley cites one report that 33 percent of patients who later disclosed their abuse, had denied it during five weeks of hospitalization at a center highly experienced in abuse treatment and sensitized to its importance.

Another of the few clear findings of the past decade is the extremely long delay that may precede disclosure even among patients in extensive therapy, reports Wooley.

She says underestimation is virtually unavoidable, yet critics express most concern with overestimation, despite lack of evidence for the latter and abundant evidence of underestimation. The accusation that the patient or therapist made it up holds sexual abuse to a test not customarily applied to clinical data, she charges.

Wooley reports that the predominantly female patients more often disclose histories of sexual abuse to female therapists. Male therapists as a whole did not realize the extent and consequences of sexual abuse until recently. Now that it is recognized, she says there is a polarization over how to deal with it in the eating disorder field. The controversy involves medical versus sociocultural models, technical vs humanistic approaches, and apolitical vs feminist analyses.

Wooley notes that the unmasking of sexual abuse at long last was largely due to the efforts of feminist writers and clinicians.

Similarly, Freud's deliberate suppression of the discovery of sexual abuse among his women patients was not revealed until the early 1980s. And it is only in the past 20 to 25 years that the social institutions that now help female victims of sexual abuse and domestic violence have developed. Until recently, childhood sexual abuse was believed to be rare and likely harmless.

Eating disorder specialists Mark Schwartz and Leigh Cohn point out that the rate of sexual abuse was estimated at only 1 in 1,000 in a major psychiatric textbook of the 1960s. But by the 1980s many publications were reporting sexual abuse of one in three females and one in seven males.

They suggest that, like Freud, male clinicians have sometimes needed not to know and not to see, in order to maintain their own illusions. "The fundamental question is: Why has it taken so long to recognize the association if, as has been reported by one major center, 80 percent of their sample of eating-disordered patients have a history of sexual abuse? Why then has there been such resistance to knowing and believing?"[27]

However, much progress has been made in the last decade in male therapists recognizing the conflicting messages adolescent girls are given in modern culture today.

Steven Levenkron, MS, author of *The Best Little Girl in the World,* suggests male therapists can be more effective if they are "parental" rather than "paternalistic" in their feelings toward patients.

"I don't think there is anything problematic about men treating women with eating disorders if they understand the dilemma many women face in today's culture. This dilemma concerns how much to value their femininity while maintaining a level of assertiveness in order to compete with men."[28]

Others say they have learned how important it is to be silent and listen to girls and women, without taking the role of "male expert."

"Many if not most of the patients we treat have been traumatized either physically, sexually or simply in relationships where they've experienced some disappointment in others," says Craig L. Johnson, a clinical psychologist and co-director of the eating disorders program at the Laureate Psychiatric Clinic in Tulsa.

This abuse information is all so new that there is wide variation in reports. Further investigation is needed to clarify the issues. What should be considered sexual abuse? How can it be assessed in a reliable way? How can experts cope with the difficulty of disclosure?

At the same time it needs to be recognized that many eating-disordered clients were not sexually or physically abused, and many sexually abused youngsters do not develop eating disorders.

Roots of eating disorders

Factors that increase a dieter's vulnerability to eating disorders are believed to be genetic, biological, psychological, sociocultural and familial, as well as a history of sexual or physical abuse.

The traditional patriarchal view holds that the roots of eating disorders lie with pathological traits of patients and their families.

But society has to take responsibility for the tremendous impact of idealizing an increasingly thin female body.

In less than two decades, the acceptable female body size has been whittled down by one-third, write Patricia Fallon, Melanie Katzman and Wooley, editors of *Feminist Perspectives on Eating Disorders.*[29] Most women no longer fit that size, and trying to do so takes up more and more of their lives. Some are pushed to an apparent point of no return by "our era's culminating demand that women give up nourishment and a large share of their bodies."

For some girls entering adolescence, accepting their rapidly-changing bodies becomes nearly impossible when placed against this cultural backdrop. Not only are their female role models extremely thin and usually dieting, but males they know are often openly denigrating large women and admiring thin women.

Complications of eating disorders

Following are mental and physical complications or traits commonly associated with anorexia nervosa and bulimia nervosa, compiled from Kaplan and Garfinkel.[30]

Mental complications

Anorexia nervosa

Many of the mental and emotional symptoms common to anorexia nervosa are directly related to the physical effects of starvation. Other traits have to do with attitudes and behavior toward eating and weight.

■ **Energy level.** Fatigue, weakness, lassitude, lethargy, apathy, decreasing energy, persistent tiredness, dizziness, faintness, light-headedness; yet compulsively exercises (hyperactive).

■ **Mood, attitude and behavior.** Moodiness, often depressed, mood swings (tyrannical); anxiety and ambivalence; irritability; critical; intolerant of others; depression; low self-esteem, self-esteem controlled through weight loss; invulnerability and success dependent on weight loss; feelings of lack of control in life; hopelessness; rigidity, highly controlled behavior; does not reveal feelings; perfectionist behavior; fantasy that weight loss can cause or prevent some life event (prevent parental divorce, attract romance); denies hunger; denies problem of weight loss (sees self as fat); denies eating disorder; body image distortion, overestimates body size and shape, "feels fat" despite emaciated appearance; ritualistic habits.

■ **Mental ability.** Inability to concentrate, decreased alertness; difficulty with reading comprehension, diminished capacity to think; loss of memory; extreme narrowing of interests; decline in ambition.

■ **Social.** Social withdrawal, isolates self from family and friends, becomes increasingly aloof and withdrawn; lonely; feelings easily hurt; avoidance by peers; worsening family relations, fights with family, cost of treatment may be a family financial drain.

■ **Weight.** Increasing preoccupation with body; frequently monitors body changes (may check with scale and/or mirror many times per day); compares size and shape to others, envious of thinner persons; heightened control, feelings of having control over body.

■ **Food, eating and hunger.** Misperception of hunger, satiety and other bodily sensations; hunger and increasing hunger; fears food and gaining weight; eats alone; guilt when eating; may secretly binge; dieting and weight increasingly important focus; unusual food-related behaviors (makes rules for specific foods, placement on plate, time of eating, size of bites, number of chews per bite); progressive preoccupation with food and eating (may begin to cook and control family eating); need to vicariously enjoy food (may collect recipes, dream of food, hoard food, enjoy watching others eat, pursue food-related careers — as dietitians, chefs, caterers).

■ **Other.** Hypersensitive to cold and heat, hypersensitive to noise and light; sleep disturbance.

Bulimia nervosa

The person with bulimia nervosa is often normal weight and may not experience the effects of starvation. However, if she has nutrition deficiencies due to purging, she may have starvation symptoms. When a patient with anorexia becomes bulimic, she or he experiences symptoms characteristic of both eating disorders.

Typically, these mental and emotional symptoms may be associated with bulimia nervosa:

■ **Mood/attitude/behavior.** Anxiety, depression; mood swings; low self-esteem, self-deprecating thoughts; embarrassment, shame related to behavior; persistent remorse; paranoid feelings; unreasonable resentments; makes excuses to go to restroom after meals; may buy large amounts of food, which suddenly disappears; impulsive as compared to anorexics who are overcontrolled.

■ **Mental ability.** Loss of ordinary willpower, poor impulse control, self-indulgent behavior; recognizes abnormal eating behavior.

■ **Social.** Depends on others for approval; feelings of isolation; unable to discuss problem, others are unhappy about food obsession; social isolation; distances self from friends and family; fear of going out in public; family, work and money problems.

■ **Weight**. Feels that self worth is dependent on low weight; constant concern with weight and body image.

■ **Food, eating and hunger.** Eats alone; eats when not hungry; preoccupation with eating and food; fears binges and eating out of control; increased dependency on bingeing; binge eating of large amount of food in a short time, feeling out of control, cannot stop eating.

■ **Purging.** Feels need to rid body of calories consumed during binge (through vomiting, laxatives, diuretics, enemas, fasting or excessive exercise); experimentation with vomiting, laxatives and diuretics often leads to regular abuse.

■ **Binge/purge cycle.** Spends much time planning, carrying out, cleaning up after bulimic episode; eliminates normal activities; complex lifestyle may develop with episodes occurring several times a day;

worsening of symptoms during times of emotional stress; feels soothed and comforted by binge/purge cycle — it may serve to relieve frustration, anxiety, anger, fear, remorse, boredom, loneliness.

■ **Other.** Dishonesty, lying; stealing food or money; drug and alcohol abuse; suicidal tendencies or attempts.

Physical complications

Anorexia nervosa

■ **Electrolytes.** May be low in potassium, sodium, chloride, calcium, magnesium, and high or low bicarbonate. Electrolyte imbalance more likely when there is dehydration and/or purging.

■ **Gastrointestinal**. Constipation is likely, may promote laxative use. Commonly there is vomiting, feelings of fullness and bloating, and abdominal discomfort. There may be ulcers, and pancreatic dysfunction. Excessive laxatives over time may result in gastrointestinal bleeding and impairment of colon functioning.

■ **Cardiovascular.** Commonly present are chest pain, arrhythmias, hypotension, edema and mitral valve prolapse. Electrocardiogram (EKG) changes. Heart rates lower than 40 beats per minute are common and as low as 25 reported in severe starvation. Prolonged QT intervals can lead to sudden death syndrome.

■ **Metabolic.** Abnormal temperature regulation and cold intolerance are common. Abnormal glucose tolerance, fasting hypoglycemia, high B-hydroxybutyric acid, high free fatty acids, hypercholesterolemia, hypercarotenemia are common. Diabetic patients with an eating disorder may have fluctuating blood glucose levels leading to serious long-term consequences.

■ **Bones.** Decreased bone mineral density may lead to fractures, growth retardation, short stature and osteoporosis.

■ **Renal.** Elevated blood urea nitrogen, changes in urinary concentration capacity, and decreased glomerular filtration rate are common.

■ **Endocrine.** Amenorrhea is 100 percent, by definition, although many anorexia nervosa patients begin to menstruate over time. Amenorrhea related to weight loss but may precede weight loss (in one-third); may cause delayed puberty, contributes to osteoporosis, breast atrophy, infertility. Hypometabolic state resulting in cold intolerance, dry skin and hair, bradycardia, constipation, fatigue, slowed reflexes. High plasma cortisol, decreased cortixol response to insulin.

■ **Hematologic.** Anemia, leukopenia, bone marrow hypocellularity, common; these effects are usually mild, but can include bleeding tendency.

- ■ **Neurological.** EEG and sleep changes are common; epileptic seizures affect up to 10 percent.
- ■ **Musculocutaneous.** Muscle weakening, muscle cramps. Hair loss, brittle hair and nails, lanugo hair, dry skin and cold extremities are common.

Bulimia nervosa

- ■ **Electrolytes.** Low potassium, low chloride, dehydration and metabolic alkalosis are common. May lead to cardiac arrest, renal failure. Dehydration is common along with hypotension, dizziness, weakness, muscle cramps. Cardiac arrhythmias affect 20 percent; unpredictable, may require emergency treatment.

  Hypochloremia is common; limits kidney's ability to excrete bicarbonate.

- ■ **Gastrointestinal.** Constipation and increased amylase common. Rarely gastric and duodenal ulcer, acute gastric dilation and rupture. Frequent abdominal pain. Severe abdominal pain may lead to rigid abdomen and shock which may result in death. Abuses of laxatives may lead to iron deficiency anemia, rectal bleeding and cathartic colon.

- ■ **Pulmonary.** Aspiration pneumonia possible from aspiration of vomitus.

- ■ **Cardiovascular.** Peripheral edema is common along with EKG changes and QT changes, which can lead to serious arrhythmias and congestive heart failure. Uncommon is sudden cardiac death. Ipecac syrup abuse may lead to death through cardiomyopathy, myocarditis.

- ■ **Metabolic.** High B-hydroxybutyric acid, free fatty acids. Less common edema, abnormal temperature regulation and cold intolerance.

- ■ **Renal.** Possible changes.

- ■ **Endocrine.** Menstrual irregularities with low body weight, dexamethasone nonsuppression common.

- ■ **Hematologic.** May be anemic with nutrition deficiency.

- ■ **Neurological.** EEG changes common. May have epileptic seizures with malnutrition and electrolyte imbalance.

- ■ **Musculocutaneous.** Calluses on dorsum of dominant hand are common from inducing gag reflex. Muscle weakening with ipecac abuse.

- ■ **Dental.** Enamel erosions with vomiting.

CHAPTER 5

Size prejudice punishes large children

■

Large children and teens often live with vicious prejudice from their classmates, parents and teachers — attitudes which can interfere with their ability to grow into self-assured, successful adults.

Size prejudice hurts people of all sizes. While it can be an actual form of child abuse for large kids, prejudice also keeps other youngsters striving to be thin enough so they'll be safe.

Research confirms what we all know, that there is strong prejudice and even oppression against obese youngsters regardless of age, sex, race and socioeconomic status. Many struggle with discrimination in education, employment, health care and social relationships.

Even young children feel the stigma of obesity and fear being a target. In one study children as young as six described silhouettes of an overweight child as "lazy, dirty, stupid, ugly, cheats and lies."

When shown drawings of a normal weight child, an overweight child, and children with various handicaps, including missing hands and facial disfigurement, children rated the overweight child as the least likable. Sadly, this bias even afflicted the larger children who felt the same prejudices.[1]

Large children and teens can be healthy, eat normally and live active lives. But the stigma may be overwhelming. It may be difficult for them to develop confident, healthy attitudes about themselves because of the devastating prejudice practiced by their peers, their parents and their teachers.

"Clearly obese children are blamed for their condition. It is an unusual person who does not fashion this into serious self-doubt and a persistent concern with dieting," says Kelly D. Brownell, an obesity researcher and professor of psychology at Yale University.[2]

Oppression against large children may evolve into a form of persecution. They are teased on the playground, called names and chosen last to play on teams.

But it is at puberty when the problems of obesity become most painful. Despite the discrimination against them, studies show that large children's sense of self-worth is similar to that of average-weight children. But in adolescence, the powerful social messages become internalized and a lifelong negative self-image can develop, according to William Dietz and Nevin Scrimshaw, in *Social Aspects of Obesity*.[3]

Gaining a strong sense of self-worth is especially difficult for large teenagers in industrially developed countries, where in recent decades both feminine and masculine ideals have become very thin. Stars of movies, television, sports and pop music are not only lean, but the males appear muscular and fit.

"All this results in a distressing position for an obese adolescent who has to face up to the negative attitudes of colleagues at school or even in the family. Clumsiness, unattractiveness to the opposite sex, are serious problems at this age," they note.

Obesity is the last socially acceptable form of prejudice, charge Albert Stunkard and Jeffery Sobal, in *Eating Disorders and Obesity:* "Obese persons remain perhaps the only group toward whom social derogation can be directed with impunity."[4]

Teachers reinforce prejudice

Discrimination has been shown in the way teachers interact with large students and the grades they give for comparable work. Acceptance into prestigious colleges is lower in one study for large females, even when they do not differ in academic qualifications, school performance or application rates to colleges.[5]

In 1993 the National Education Association launched an investigation into size discrimination against students and teachers in the schools as a human rights and civil rights issue. This is the nation's largest teacher organization — the professionals who see the worst examples of size prejudice daily and potentially have the power to bring about change.

The next year NEA published its 27-page "Report on Size Discrimination," which describes size discrimination in schools at every level.[6]

The report says the school experience is one of "ongoing prejudice, unnoticed discrimination and almost constant harassment" for large students, and "socially acceptable yet outrageous insensitivity and rudeness" for large teachers.

"At the elementary level, children learn that it is acceptable to dislike and deride fatness. From nursery school through college, fat students experience ostracism, discouragement, and sometimes violence. Often ridiculed by their peers and discouraged by even well-meaning education employees, fat students develop low self-esteem and have limited horizons. They are deprived of places on honor rolls, sports teams, and cheerleading squads and are denied letters of recommendation."

A member of the investigating team sympathized with large teens who are uncomfortable in showers and don't want other students to stare at or ridicule them. Another told of a high school drill team that for 10 years excluded overweight girls from the team. Those who were progressing toward their goal weight were allowed to practice at school but not perform in public.

My friend Carol Johnson, a Wisconsin therapist who founded Largely Positive support groups for large women, writes in her book, *Self-Esteem Comes in All Sizes,* how her cheerleading ambitions came to an abrupt end.[7]

"One of my dreams was to be a cheerleader. When tryouts were announced in the seventh grade, I signed up immediately and practiced night and day. After tryouts, I knew I had given a flawless performance. However, the physical education teacher who was judging the competition took me aside and gently told me that although I was one of the best candidates, she simply could not choose me. The reason? I was too chubby. My body was unacceptable for public display.

"Shortly thereafter, I became intrigued by the baton and decided to take twirling lessons. You would have thought the cheerleader episode would have deterred me forever, but somehow it didn't. I dreamed of leading the marching band down the football field, and adept as I was, I thought there was good chance this dream would become reality. Reality did set in, but not the one I had dreamed about. Once again I was trying to do something chubby girls weren't supposed to do — put themselves on display. This time I was told not to bother because the uniforms wouldn't fit me. I didn't even try out. And the message pierced deeper: You're not acceptable.

"The truth is that my weight in high school exceeded the weight charts by no more than 30 pounds. Now, when I look at my high school pictures, I don't think I look at all heavy. Yet at the time those extra 30 pounds felt like the weight of the world on my shoulders. Losing weight had become the most important thing in my life."

Carol says her parents were always loving, supportive and proud of her, but they couldn't protect her from the outside world. "I truly believed, deep in my heart that I was not as good as the thinner girls. Only by losing weight could I become their equal."

The NEA report quotes a *New York Times* article about a girl named Aleta Walker as an example of the "outrageous behavior" to which large children are subjected in schools.

Aleta never had any friends during her childhood and adolescence in Hannibal, Mo. Instead she was ridiculed and bullied every day. When she walked down the halls at school, boys would flatten themselves against the lockers and cry, "Wide load!"

But the worst was lunchtime, she said. "Every day there was this production of watching me eat lunch." She tried to avoid going to the school cafeteria. "I would hide out in the bathroom. I would hide out behind the gym by the baseball diamond. I would hide in the library."

One day, schoolmates started throwing food at her as she sat at lunch. Plates of spaghetti splashed onto her face, and the long greasy strands dripped onto her clothes.

"Everyone was laughing and pointing. They were making pig noises. I just sat there," she said.

Another friend of mine through the size acceptance movement is Cheri Erdman, now a 42-year-old therapist and college teacher. She was actually sent away from home at age 5, on the advice of a kindergarten teacher, to live for more than a year in a residential weight treatment facility for children with "special nutritional needs." In her book, *Nothing to Lose: A Guide to Sane Living in a Larger Body,* Erdman, describes the sadness of being separated from her family for so long.[8]

Echoes from his youth, writes Dan Davis of Salinas, Calif., in *Radiance,* are the shouts: "I don't want you on my team. You're too fat to run." "Look at the fat tub." "You're belly looks like a watermelon."

Today he says, "My stomach still knots when I remember . . . I'll carry the scars to my grave. (But) today's kids have it worse."[9]

No safe haven at home

For some children, fat oppression, teasing and ridicule comes from inside the family circle, so there is no escape from tormentors.

Pat, 34, describes her father's disdain of her size in *Real Women Don't Diet.* "My experience of prejudice for being fat started at a very young age. The sadness and teasing I went through then was not from individuals outside my family; it was from within my family, by the people who are supposed to most love you. At the age of 9, I did not consider myself overweight, but in my father's opinion I was not only overweight but also a 'fat cow' and a 'fat pig.' His ridicule and teasing continued to tolerate the hatefulness of my classmates calling me 'fat Pat,' but then I would go home and hear my father threaten to send me to Missouri. He wanted to have his mom lock me up and feed me bread and water so that I could lose weight.

"My father's threats were always at the tip of his tongue. One time he had a new idea: 'If I tie you to the back of my truck and make you run around the block a few times, you'll really lose weight.' Although he never did it, just the horror of knowing it might happen was never far away. During all the years of growing up, I never was able to defend myself. I felt like I was a leper or something very bad, just for being overweight. I spent years taking drugs. I overdosed many times. Why should I care? My life wasn't worth that much. After all, I was different. I was fat."[10]

Effects of this stigma carry over into adulthood, especially for women, reports Dietz.

Women who are overweight as adolescents or young adults earn less, are less likely to marry, complete fewer years of school, and have higher rates of poverty than their normal weight peers. Fewer of these effects occur for overweight males.[11]

One study shows adults who were overweight as children, but of normal weight as adolescents, had a body image comparable to that of individuals who had never been overweight. But adults who had been obese as adolescents had an extremely negative body image and feelings of low self-worth.

Some of them experience a great deal of unresolved anger and rage. Jean Rubel, 36, describes turning this anger against herself.

"Under my loneliness simmered a lake of molten rage. Sometimes I turned it loose when I felt ignored, criticized, misunderstood, or unloved. Most of the time, though, I held it in the pit of my stomach, where it became the only defense I could find against my belief that I was flawed in some critical way that kept me from joining the human race. Unfortunately, I too often turned this hateful energy against myself in storms of self-criticism and loathing. I began to blame my body for all my problems. If I weren't so ugly, so big, so soft and flabby, I would be happy and popular. I was six feet tall and 145 pounds. According to yearbook pictures I was slender and reasonably attractive, but I couldn't see it. I wanted to be thin, admired, and loved. Instead I felt awkward, shy, fat, defective and extremely lonely."[12]

Too much pain

Life can hold a lot of pain and humiliation for some large kids. At times it may seem unbearable.

The Fort Lauderdale Sun-Sentinel in Florida reported a tragedy on August 27, 1996, that took place the day before school opened in the fall.[13]

To 12-year-old Samuel John Graham, starting at the new middle school meant being called fat and getting teased by kids again. Broward County Sheriff's detectives said Samuel so dreaded the idea of walking into the first day of classes on Monday that he got up in the middle of the night and hanged himself from a tree in the back of his Fort Lauderdale-area home.

As they got ready for the first day of school, his younger brothers, 8 and 10, looked outside and saw Samuel hanging by a rope from a tree. They called their father, who cut his son down, called paramedics, and tried to resuscitate him, but it was no use. He was pronounced dead at the scene, and his father went out and chopped down the tree his eldest son had used to take his life.

The last time the family saw Samuel was about 10:30 Sunday evening, when they prayed together. Then Samuel went to bed. At 2:30 Monday morning, his grandmother heard Samuel stirring and thought he had gotten up for a snack, according to the report. They found a flashlight and step-stool beside his body the next morning.

Samuel, 5-feet-4, 174 pounds, had talked of suicide before and his humiliation at the teasing from kids at school. He was sensitive, and when they chased him down the street or smacked the back of his head, he sometimes cried. A reporter observed that photos in the family living room showed him as the fat kid, who didn't have any friends. "The easy target. The mark. It's all there in his eyes: The sweetness. The shyness. The hurt."

His parents tried. They met with his teachers, showered him with affection and love, took him to physicians and counsellors, sent him to Jamaica that summer to spend time with an uncle, a fitness buff, hoping he would build muscle and self-esteem. Now they are setting up a center for shy, overweight children, where they can swim without shame. Sammy loved to swim, they said, but only after dark. He was too ashamed to let anyone see him in his bathing suit.

Headlines two or three years earlier reported another boy tormented by his elementary school peers, who shot and killed himself in the classroom in front of those who had ridiculed him.

Invisible behind a stony mask

Charisse Goodman recounts the unfairness of her childhood experiences in *The Invisible Woman*.[14]

"I was always 'the fat kid.' I wasn't me. I wasn't a name or a person, just an object described by an adjective. If I was naturally shy, I became doubly so.

"To make things worse, my family moved several times during my childhood. I found out early that I'd be lucky to have one or two friends who didn't care what I looked like. I learned that no matter what anyone says, it really doesn't count if you're smart, kind, funny, sweet, generous, or caring because if you also happen to be heavy, you may find yourself on the receiving end of more cruelty than you even knew existed.

"I learned that keeping to myself and minding my own business didn't help because people would seek me out to ridicule and humiliate me. I learned that 'ignoring it,' as I was nonchalantly advised to do by my emotionally disengaged parents, usually just made me a greater challenge to bullies, so that I inevitably became 'the one to get.' I learned that adults are often indifferent to the suffering of a fat child, perhaps because on some level they agree with her tormentors, or maybe it's just convenient for them to believe that an abused child will somehow emerge unscathed into adulthood, magically free of emotional scars.

"I discovered that anytime I moved my body, people would laugh at me, and that even if I sat still and quietly read a book they would point and laugh. I learned that if they saw me cry or show any weakness, they would laugh at me even more. And so I learned to cry alone, and laugh alone, and live alone inside my head. I learned that the word 'pretty' never included me.

"Even those times when I lost weight to try and fit in, it was never enough, and I grew to realize that when it was time to choose teammates for a game, or dates for a dance, I was invisible; but when someone needed a cheap laugh or a quick ego boost at my expense, people saw me, all right. I learned my place. I tried to learn not to care.

"As I grew up, I assumed a stone-faced mask in order to deprive people of their sickening delight in hurting me, a mask which in later years I would find extremely difficult to remove. I became a tense child with a perpetual air of bewilderment. But I was not angry. Any anger on my part was met by adults with the huffy insistence that I had a hostility problem. What other people did to me was natural and normal, while I was neither.

"Now I am a grown woman. I know without a doubt that in every town and every city, in every state in America, countless other fat children are learning the same heartbreaking, soul-destroying lessons that I was forced to learn. My pain and the pain of others like me has been conveniently invisible to thin people for far too long. They have been too comfortable with the price that we have paid for their imaginary superiority.

"At long last, I am angry."

Venting feelings

Nancy Summer, another friend and leader in the size acceptance movement, brings workshops in anti-violence, anti-prejudice programs to sixth-grade girls in schools.[15]

She encourages the girls to vent their worst prejudices against large people and get all the negative things out in the open right away.

"I invite them to insult me. 'What do you think when you see a person as fat as me? What words come to mind? You can be honest.' (I weigh more than 400 pounds.)

"After the initial giggling and squirming in chairs, the responses are never the same. In one class, a rambunctious thin girl looks me dead in the eye and calls me a horse! 'Good!' I say. I smile and write horse on the flip chart and then ask if they can think of other animals that are associated with fat people. Soon horse is joined by suggestions from other girls: cow, elephant, pig, hippo, buffalo and whale. Then we discuss how beautiful these animals are in their own right. My calm response to the challenge sets the tone for that workshop.

"Whether the girls are polite or candid, aware of the issues or not, we always manage to bring out many of the stereotypes and negative language that they've heard (and use) about fat people. They especially enjoy talking about their larger teachers in a setting where they can 'get away with it.' One girl actually admits that she teased a teacher until she made her cry. She is proud of this revelation until she hears her classmates define this as being mean.

"When a group is too polite, I ask what the boys say to or about fat girls, and that often brings lots of responses: 'Shamu,' 'bubble butt,' and 'lard ass' are favorites. We also discuss the many stereotypes people believe about fat kids and adults. 'Fat and lazy,' 'Fat people eat all the time,' and 'Boys don't think fat girls are pretty,' are just some of the responses I get.

"I always counter the negative stereotypes with facts and personal stories. For example, when one girl says that fat people are stupid, I counter with the fact that when I was in sixth grade, I was invited into a program where I could skip eighth grade.

"But always I stress my basic message: bias against fat hurts people of all sizes. 'Imagine that you are sitting in the lunchroom and a bully starts making fun of a fat kid a few tables away. How does that make you feel?' I ask them. 'We can imagine that the fat kid feels bad about being picked on, but what about all the other kids who hear it?'

"'I'd be afraid he'd pick on me next,' one girl responds. Another says, 'I'd be afraid that if I got fat, people would pick on me, too.' 'I wouldn't eat my dessert.' 'I'd probably laugh, too,' one candid soul admits, but goes on to tell us about a fat boy in her school who always laughs when people pick on him. One brave girl says, 'I'd tell him to shut up.'

"I explain that it isn't just large kids and adults who are hurt by size discrimination. Everyone else is hurt, too, because as long as fat is hated, everyone will be afraid of becoming fat. Fear of fat makes everyone unhappy and dissatisfied with their bodies. And that makes us have lower self-esteem and less self-confidence. And sometimes it can lead to dangerous diets and eating disorders."

Clearly size prejudice is a potent force for these youngsters and sixth grade girls understand it well.

CHAPTER 6

Overweight rates
keep rising

■

When is a child overweight? What causes it? And what can we do about it?

These are old questions and yet ones so new that before 1980, many believed obesity to be simply a problem of too many calories. As a result, the solutions offered by experts were often simplistic — and claimed to be effective even when they weren't.

Scientists around the world are studying these urgent questions and many others: What are the hallmarks of obesity? Does it start in childhood through excess fat cell development, or even in the womb? Is it most likely to be triggered at high-risk points during a child's development? How powerful are genetic factors? And if heredity is the important determining factor, why are we seeing such steep increases in childhood obesity in just the past decade?

While there have been advances, much remains unknown and the subject of intense debate. The bottom line is that researchers and many health professionals now recognize obesity as a complex condition that resists intervention. The fact is, there is much we don't know about childhood obesity — or what to do about it.

"Obesity continues to humble the scientific community by eluding effective understanding and intervention in many important respects," says Shiriki Kumanyika, associate professor of nutrition epidemiology at Pennsylvania State University.[1]

Prevalence

While researchers and health professionals ponder childhood overweight, its causes and outcomes, one thing is clear: The prevalence has increased sharply in the last decade for both children and adolescents in the U.S. Not only are more youngsters overweight, but they are more severely overweight than ever before.

The landmark study revealing this striking new evidence is the Third National Health and Nutrition Examination Study which gathered measurement data from 1988-1994 in two three-year phases. This study looked at a national sampling of 8,534 youth ages 6 to 17, and compared their weight with children measured in 1963. It's one of the most comprehensive studies of American youth, done by researchers at the National Center for Health Statistics at the Centers for Disease Control and Prevention in Hyattsville, Md.[2]

Figure 1

Overweight definition

at the 95th percentile

Age (years)	BOYS		GIRLS	
	Height (inches)	Weight (pounds)	Height (inches)	Weight (pounds)
6	47	56	47	57
8	51	75	52	80
10	56	96	56	104
12	60	123	61	137
14	66	164	63	151
16	69	183	65	173

Average height and weight that meets the definition of overweight originally set at the 95th percentile. Overweight is defined as at or above this level.[1]

NHANES III/AFRAID TO EAT 1997

To define the cutoff point for overweight, the researchers used the 95th percentile of body mass index, as set in the 1960s. This means 5 percent of youngsters were overweight at that time, by definition. Weight for height at the 95th percentile is given for each age in *figure 1*. This is a more conservative definition than the 85th percentile, which is sometimes used, and finds fewer kids overweight, but is preferable because it is less likely to include and stigmatize children who don't belong in the overweight category because of growth and puberty fat changes.

Using this definition, 14 percent of children age 6 to 11, and 12 percent of adolescents age 12 to 17 are overweight in the NHANES III study. This is a big increase compared with 5 percent in the 1960s, and most of it came during the last decade (*figure 2*).

Phase 1 of the study identified about 22 percent of youth (12 to 17) as being at the 85 percent level. This is the level used by Healthy People 2000 in setting the goal that 15 percent or less of children and

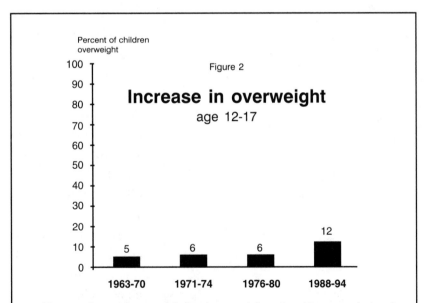

Percent of children overweight

Figure 2

Increase in overweight
age 12-17

The prevalence of overweight has increased from 5 to 12 percent during the last three decades for boys and girls age 12-17, at the 95th percentile. Most of the increase came during the last decade. NHANES III (1988-1994).[2]

ARCH PEDIATR ADOLESC MED 1995; MMWR 1997
NHANES III/AFRAID TO EAT 1997

adolescents would be overweight by the year 2000. This goal is now regarded as impossible, and all trends are in the opposite direction. Cutoff points at the 85th percentile fall at a BMI of 23 for ages 12 to 14, 24 for ages 15 to 17, and 26 for ages 18 to 19.

A closer analysis shows that this weight increase is not consistent at all levels. The most increase comes at the upper end. In other words, the heaviest children are now heavier than children in earlier studies — and more of them have moved above the cutoff point. At the other levels percentages have remained fairly constant for the past three decades.[3]

What alarms public health officials is that rates of overweight were fairly stable for children and teens during the 1960s and 1970s, but since the early 1980s, both children and adults have gained weight, particularly at the upper end. The number of overweight adults has increased from about 25

Figure 3

Prevalence of overweight

by sex, age and race/ethnicity[3]

Boys	95th percentile
6-11	
Total	14.7
White, non-Hispanic	13.2
Black, non-Hispanic	14.7
Mexican American	18.8
12-17	
Total	12.3
White, non-Hispanic	11.6
Black, non-Hispanic	12.5
Mexican American	15.0
Girls	
6-11	
Total	12.5
White, non-Hispanic	11.9
Black, non-Hispanic	17.9
Mexican American	15.8
12-17	
Total	10.7
White, non-Hispanic	9.6
Black, non-Hispanic	16.3
Mexican American	14.0

NHANES III/AFRAID TO EAT 1997

to 34 percent during the same period.

Another study that documents increases in overweight for children is the long-term Bogalusa Heart Study. During 14 years, this survey of 2,500 to 3,500 youth measured dramatic increases in overweight for ages 5 to 14.[4] At each age level, children were heavier by 5.5 pounds in 1984 than in 1973. However, again percentages at the lean and average weights tended to remain consistent, while most increases came in the heavier categories. Yet the researchers couldn't find that the heavier children were eating more calories than leaner children.

Higher rates for minorities

The NHANES III study finds more minority children overweight than white children at all ages *(figure 3)*.

Black children tend to be taller, heavier, and to mature earlier. Even at age 10, black girls were 11 pounds heavier, 1.6 inches taller, had more body fat, and reached puberty earlier than white girls, in a study of black Harlem youth.[5]

Overweight prevalence is also high for American Indian children. Rates range up to 40 or 50 percent, depending on the study, definition and tribe.[6] A look at Zuni children found that more than half of girls and one third of boys ages 11 to 20 were overweight. Interestingly, a study of Cherokee teens found that gender trend reversed — half of boys and one-fourth of girls were overweight.[7]

The Pima, who suffer extremely high rates of type II diabetes associated with obesity, also tend to have children who are taller, heavier and have more body fat than white children the same age. One study of Pima youth shows about half exceed the 95th percentile of body mass index.[8]

Fat patterning and body composition

Fat distribution can indicate if children may be at risk for health problems later in life. When excess fat is concentrated on the upper body or abdomen, in a centralized pattern (apple shape), rather than in the lower body (pear shape), they have a greater tendency to develop risk factors related to heart disease and diabetes.[9]

Inherited factors including race/ethnicity may determine a child's
build and fat patterning. Black and Mexican American children tend
to have more upper body fat than white children, and this increases
with age, particularly for boys, according to William Mueller of the
School of Public Health, University of Texas Health Science Center
who analyzed data from national studies.[10]

Defining obesity

Currently, there is no accepted definition of obesity or overweight
for children and adolescents. It may be defined by BMI, percentile
cutoff points, or percent body fat (sometimes 25 percent body fat for
boys and 30 percent for girls).[11]

But today many specialists are saying other factors need to be
considered, such as family history to determine what may be normal
for a particular child. Whether because of genetics or family practices, the assessment of obesity must involve the family as well as the
individual youngster, says the California position paper *Children and
Weight: A Changing Perspective,* by Eileen B. Peck, DrPH, RD, and
Helen D. Ullrich, MA, RD.

"Do we really need a definition of childhood obesity?" asks
Katherine M. Flegal, PhD, Chief Medical Statistics Branch, Division
of Health Examination at the National Center for Health Statistics.

Putting children in categories by level of overweight will stigmatize them. That's why Flegal and the other federal researchers reporting NHANES III findings are reluctant to set a cutoff that labels
children, and why they finally set it only at the 95th percentile. They're
concerned their statistics will be used aggressively in dealing with
obesity in youth. Children grow and develop at every age in widely
differing ways, they remind health providers.[12]

The terms overweight and obesity are often used interchangeably,
as they are in this book, here defined in a general way as any recognized degree of excess weight or body fat.

What happened?

Although we knew it was coming from many smaller studies all
pointing to increases in overweight, the new nationwide statistics sent

a shock wave through the health community.

What happened? Why did obesity rates jump across the board for young and old, males and females, and for every ethnic and racial group during the last decade?

Perhaps the simplest explanation is that children are less active. Another answer is too much high-fat food or too many calories, and certainly this is a likely factor for many youth today. Yet, on the average, children as well as adults are eating less fat today than a decade ago, and calorie increases, if any, appear to be small. Fat consumption has dropped from 36 to 34 percent of total calories in the last decade. Some specialists question whether dietary changes and the decrease in fat itself may be part of the problem.

Other possible factors: Women are having bigger babies today, encouraged to gain more weight in pregnancy by public health policies aimed at preventing low birth weight, especially in minorities — and this may increase the legacy of overweight for both babies and teenage mothers. Also, there may be higher population increases in groups with the "thrifty gene."

The nature of obesity is not well understood. The interplay of genetics, food supply, physical activity, culture, socioeconomic and psychological factors all have a profound effect on the regulation of appetite, satiety, and how calories are used — or stored as fat.

The tendency to gain excessive fatness varies from one person to another, even in the same family, and even when food intake, physical activity and lifestyle appear to be the same. Metabolism may play a part, but it is much more complex than this. It is likely that genetic factors route more fat into storage for some individuals, and that they have extraordinary ability to protect that stored fat and restore it quickly after being depleted from dieting or starvation.

Genetic factors

Family makes a difference in two ways. About 25 percent of adult obesity can be traced to genetic origin and another 30 percent to family cultural factors, according to Claude Bouchard, PhD, a professor of exercise physiology at Laval University, Quebec, who has done extensive research comparing identical twins, reared apart

Ethnic differences in fat patterning

Ethnic differences in body build and fat patterning were analyzed by William Mueller of the School of Public Health, University of Texas Health Science Center, using data on national and other studies of children and adolescents. His studies show ethnicity accounts for about one-third to one-half of the variance of sex and maturation. His findings are independent of average fatness levels. However, Mueller suggests some of the variance may be the result of the differing obesity levels in black and Mexican American children.

Comparing statistics on black, Mexican American and white children, he reports the following:

1. Children, ages 1 to 5
- Preschool children are much more peripheral in fat distribution (less centralized) than older children.
- Black preschool children have more centralized or upper body fat patterning than white preschoolers.

2. Adolescents
- Mexican American children have higher skinfold measures at triceps, subscapular and suprailiac, but lower at medial calf site, compared with white children; thus, theirs is a centralized obesity.
- Black children have lower skinfolds at both arm and leg sites than white children; their fat is more centrally distributed.

3. Girls, ages 12 to 17
- Black and Mexican American girls have a more central distribution of fat than white girls.

- Fatness increases with age for all three groups.

4. Boys, ages 12 to 17
- Centrality of fat increases with age in all three groups.
- Black and Mexican American boys have a more centralized fat patterning than white boys.

5. Other differences, ages 6 to 17
- Black children tend to have more centralized fat patterning at all ages, with less arm and leg fat, compared with white children.
- Black children have the broadest shoulders and narrowest hips, compared with Mexican and white children.
- Mexican American children have more upper body fatness with less leg fat, compared with white children.
- Mexican Americans tend to have the narrowest shoulders of the three groups.
- A sex difference emerges at puberty, but ethnic differences remain.
- Individuals with non-insulin dependent diabetes (ages 14 to 17) tend to have broader shoulders and narrower hips than nondiabetic youth of same sex and age.
- Circumference ratios of waist-to-hip show less ethnic difference than skinfolds, yet show consistent sex difference. Thus circumferences may be measuring muscle and bone development, not fatness levels.[4]

Bouchard, Johnston, 1988
Healthy Weight Journal, 1988
AFRAID TO EAT 1997

and together, adoptees and their two sets of families, and nine types of relatives.[13]

A child with two overweight parents has an 80 percent chance of becoming overweight, in one analysis, compared with 14 percent for the child of two normal weight parents.[14]

The "thrifty gene" theory helps explain why obesity rates are so high for children of African, American Indian, Mexican or Pacific Island descent. This theory holds that certain traits helped early humans survive under starving conditions in ancient times. People with these thrifty traits were most likely to survive, have children and pass on these genes. The closer modern people are to their subsistence roots, the more likely they retain the thrifty gene, while those of us whose ancestors came from agricultural areas and overcame starvation conditions may have lost it.

Thus, the thrifty gene is like driving a highly efficient sports car with excellent gas mileage, compared with an old "gas guzzler" that requires and wastes much fuel. In primitive times, having an efficient gene was beneficial, but in our modern world of abundant high-fat food and sedentary living, it's a problem that easily promotes obesity.[15]

It's quite clear that genetic factors can affect such regulators as metabolism, thermogenesis, endocrine function, fat storage, appetite and satiety. Still, Bouchard cautions against putting too much blame on genetics. Many factors are involved, and there's "a lot of chaos in the body system we're working with," he says. "We are probably overemphasizing the importance of genetics in obesity . . . We are seeing big increases in obesity worldwide — this has to be the result of environmental factors."

Inactivity

It's hard to measure physical activity, but most experts agree there's probably been a continuing decline in activity.

Our streets are perceived as unsafe, and whether this is a determining factor or not, more children and youth stay indoors, watching television, playing video games and surfing the Internet. In today's climate of decreasing budgets, thousands of schools are cutting physical education programs. In 1995 only 25 percent of school children attended daily physical education class.

The more children watch television, the higher their risk for becoming overweight, no matter what their race, according to some studies. This may mean they are less active or snack more in front of the small screen, or that television itself may have a lulling effect by lowering metabolism, as one study found.

Children spent more time watching television during the 1980s than ever before, and at the same time overweight increased. In one study of the relationship between television and weight, which may also explain some racial differences, black girls watched an average of 36 hours a week compared with 24 hours for white girls. They were also more overweight, as were girls of both races who watched more television. Girls who said they usually ate while watching television consumed more calories than others. And almost twice as many black girls as white girls reported that they usually ate while watching television.[16]

Food intake

The kinds of food children are eating may also make a difference. Today kids eat more foods like crackers, chips, dessert foods and candy — and less meat, eggs and milk, which may provide more satisfaction.

In one large study, black and white girls ages 9 and 10 kept food diaries for three days, providing insight into the link between body composition, eating and exercise. The black girls tended to be heavier, and ate more calories and fat than the white girls. They ate less meat, milk and cheese and snacked more on high-fat foods. They also watched more hours of television and videos per week — and it was this factor that seemed most directly related to overweight. For white girls, eating high-fat foods and watching TV were both associated with overweight.[17]

Eating patterns have changed, too. Children are eating fewer regular meals, fewer meals at home, and fewer meals with family. They eat more outside the home, often at fast-food restaurants in which increasingly larger meals are being served.

Family control effects

What you do, what you say and how you eat in a family counts. Simple things, like urging a child to clean her plate can have a direct effect on overweight.

Fourteen families with children ages 1 to 3 were observed at meals over time in a psychology study at North Dakota State University in Fargo. The researchers found that the overweight children were urged both verbally and nonverbally to eat more by their parent over twice as often as normal weight children. Overweight children received an average of 43 prompts per meal compared with 18 for the normal weight children *(figure 4)*. All children usually ate more when prompted to do so. Parents prompted their children to eat with words or by giving them food one-fourth of the time. When children refused, almost 90 percent of the time parents encouraged them to eat, and 70 percent of the time they did.

The researchers concluded many parents selectively encourage eating in their very young children in ways that override satiety signals and may lead to excess weight gain.[18]

On the other hand, children may also gain excess weight from being underfed and encouraged to eat less than satisfies their needs, reports Ellyn Satter. She says parents often believe their children can't regulate food intake and it's their job as parent to get children to eat. But those strategies, intended to feed a child a well-balanced diet, can be coercive and controlling. Studies suggest that very young children can indeed regulate their own food intake, and that a controlling, authoritarian parenting style impedes their ability to develop self-control, she says.[19]

When parents focus too much on what to eat, when to eat, or how much food is left on the plate, their children don't learn normal eating habits of responding to hunger and satiety. The parent who is dieting may be overconcerned about the child's weight and eating.

Poor family communication may also contribute to overweight. If children are isolated in a disinterested or disengaged family, they may be at a higher risk of overweight, reports Laurel Mellin, MA, RD, San Francisco. Her study of 254 obese adolescents found that four factors accounted for most of the weight differences: family cohesion, adolescent communication, age of obesity onset and the mother's weight. Surprisingly, the major environmental factors were not diet and activity, but instead were related to relationships, family cohesion and communication. Obesity increased for children as families were less engaged and the adolescent less engaging. Mellin suggests that targeting family communication and teaching family interactional skills may be more effective in preventing obesity than just targeting diet and physical activity.[20]

How obesity develops in infants

From birth, babies born to overweight mothers seem at higher risk for becoming overweight. Studies of British and Canadian children show that even if the babies are normal weight at birth, by age 6 months they are growing faster and are heavier than other infants. However not all fat babies are at risk.[21]

Some researchers have observed that infants who are quiet, inactive and placid tend to become overweight even with moderate intakes of food. This may be considered normal.

A child's family, eating habits and activity, but not necessarily food intake, seem to determine whether a baby will grow into an

---

Figure 4

Parental food prompts
per meal[5]

Average per child	Normal weight child	Overweight child
Encouragements to eat	4	16
Food presentations	11	20
Offers of food	3	7
Total food prompts	18	43

KLESGES/HEALTHY WEIGHT JOURNAL/ION REVIEWS 1988

overweight child.

Infant feeding

Breastfeeding seems to be a healthy course for both mothers and babies, but its association with weight gain is unclear. Some studies in the 1970s suggested that bottle-feeding and the early introduction of solid foods contributed to childhood obesity, but more recent studies refute that claim.

A 16-year longitudinal study followed 180 children from age 6 months to age 16, in Berkeley, Calif. The type of infant feeding or when solid food was introduced made no difference. Neither did the kinds of food eaten for meals or snacks, or whether the child had a sweet tooth.[22]

A four-year study of babies in Maine found no relationship between formula feeding or the early introduction of solid foods and preschool obesity. Solid foods were given earlier to babies who were bottle-fed, while babies who were breast-fed started solid foods later. After four years, 12 percent of the children were considered overweight, with no relationship to these feeding practices.[23]

Bigger babies

Since 1989, U.S. Public Health directives have called on women to produce larger babies that average 8 to 8.5 pounds by gaining more weight in pregnancy, in a move to reduce the number of small, premature babies. Yet there is evidence to suggest that larger babies are more likely to be overweight later in life, especially for minority children. And gaining more weight in pregnancy clearly increases obesity risk for mothers.

Ray Yip, MD, MPH, Centers for Disease Control, reports that CDC surveillance programs show birth weight influences later growth: heavy babies are four times as likely to become heavy 5-year-olds.[24]

Another federal analysis of height and weight at age 6 to 11 showed similar results: children with higher birth weights were heavier and taller. Increased early height is related to earlier maturity, which in turn is related to obesity.[25]

Weight gain in pregnancy

Girls with higher levels of body fat enter puberty earlier, increasing their risk for overweight and for early pregnancy. During pregnancy these early teen and preteen mothers are being urged by public health policy to have heavier babies. Low-income girls and those from ethnic groups with high obesity rates face even more risk. Having more pregnancies is also linked to obesity.

Women have long recognized that excess weight gain in pregnancy is critical in triggering obesity, but it is still being largely ignored by the medical and health communities. Many doctors shrug off such concerns, saying any excess weight can be taken off later. Unfortunately, this is not true.

The problem of excessive weight gain in pregnancy is especially acute for racial and ethnic minorities. There is evidence that it is normal for African-American women to gain less in pregnancy than white women and have smaller babies, who then grow faster in their early years than white babies. By age 1 to 4, growth is accelerated for black children over that of white children, according to Kumanyika. Small babies are common in Africa, she says.[26]

American Indian babies, too, were known to be smaller in earlier times and childbirth was easier. This may be another genetic survival trait. The insistence of health officials that minority babies be large may not be as beneficial as hoped — certainly it is paralleled by a steep increase in obesity for both minority women and their children.

At the same time, many young pregnant girls are so poorly nourished, often from dieting, that they do not gain enough weight to support both a healthy growth of the infant and their own growth needs. Young girls have high rates of giving birth to very small, high-risk, premature babies. Thus, it is important that pregnant teens and preteens get early nutrition counseling and prenatal care.

Risks of overweight

Overweight children may be at increased risk for diabetes and cardiovascular problems tracking into adulthood. And since the social stigma of being large is so strong, they're also at increased risk of using dangerous weight loss methods or developing eating disorders.

Increasingly, health problems from hazardous weight loss attempts and ill-advised treatment are being recognized as risks of being overweight for children as well as adults.

Health risks related specifically to adolescent obesity, as given by Pauline Powers, MD, at the NIH Strategy Development Workshop for Public Education on Weight and Obesity, include:

- Increased blood pressure.
- Increased total cholesterol and abnormal lipoprotein rations.
- Hyperinsulineamia.[27]

It should be noted that physical fitness is related to blood pressure in 5- and 6-year-old children, independent of obesity, in both cross-sectional and longitudinal studies, says Steven Shea, MD, Columbia Presbyterian Medical Center. Because of mobility or social reasons, some large children tend to be sedentary, which can increase these problems or even be the root cause, rather than obesity.

Being overweight as a child may influence adult health. For men, Tufts University researchers found those who were 20 pounds or more overweight as teenagers were twice as likely as those of normal weight to have died or have heart disease by age 70. They were also more likely to suffer colon and rectal cancer and to develop gout. Men who had been overweight as teens but not as adults had lower risk.

However, for women who had been overweight as teens there was no added health risk at age 70. They did have double the risk of arthritis and eight times as much difficulty in walking a quarter of a mile, climbing stairs and lifting heavy objects. The study looked at health records of students and tracked their weights and health for 55 years.[28]

In the Bogalusa Heart Study, a clustering of three risk factors correlate highly with obesity, especially centralized obesity: systolic blood pressure, fasting insulin, and ratio of low and very low density lipoprotein cholesterol to high density lipoprotein cholesterol (the "bad" vs "good" cholesterol). Children in the upper third weight category showed increased clustering of these factors, compared with lean children. The Bogalusa team suggests preventing obesity early in life may be important in reducing heart disease later on.[29]

Powers also suggests these psychological risks:

- Poor body image, "imprinted" in adolescence.
- Low self-esteem, including fear of obesity and increasing preoccupation with size and shape.
- Cultural stigmatization — both children and adults devalue overweight children.

Some childhood specialists suggest the biggest problems of childhood obesity may be emotional and psychological, being labelled and stigmatized as obese, long-term damage to self-esteem and body concept.[30] It is clear obesity can be a severe social handicap.

Yet others point out that, while this is true, cultural stigma is not a reason to change the child, but rather to change the culture.

Early puberty

Early puberty is another, largely-unrecognized risk of obesity. It's a factor in the high rates of preteen pregnancy in the U.S. and increases the risk of reproductive cancers later in life, writes Rose Frisch, PhD, Harvard Center for Population Studies, in *Adipose Tissue and Reproduction*.[31]

The age of puberty for American and European boys and girls has dropped steadily during the last 100 years. Instead of reaching menarche at age 15 or 16 and their adult height at 20 to 21 years as they did 100 years ago, American girls now reach menarche at an average of 12.8 years and complete growth by age 16 to 18, according to Frisch's research.

Why is this happening?

Frisch suggests this trend is related to higher body fat and inactivity. Girls need about 22 percent body fat to reach menarche, she says, and mean weight at puberty is 105 pounds. Average body fat for young women is 25 to 30 percent, according to the American Alliance for Health, Physical Education, Recreation and Dance, 1984.

"Children now are bigger sooner. And girls on the average reach the mean weight at menarche . . . more quickly," says Frisch.

Female athletes still average 15.5 years at menarche, about the same as a century ago. Girls and young women who exercise or train athletically can delay puberty by months or even years. In a study of female college athletes who began training before menarche, the average began having their periods about three years later than women who began training after menarche, Frisch says.

At the same time, it is critical that female athletes eat well and be fully nourished to avoid risk of fragile bones and stress fractures.

Tracking obesity

One of the more controversial issues in determining what to do about childhood obesity is its impact on later life.

Does obesity track into adulthood? Is an overweight child charting a course that will lead to lifelong obesity and perhaps related health risks, which could be altered by making early changes?

Or will young children outgrow their fatness? If they do, being wrongly identified as obese may contribute to psychosocial difficulties. Growth may also be affected by weight loss attempts.

Two important factors to consider are the severity and age of the youngster. Severe obesity at any age is probably likely to continue. Yet it is important to recognize that most large infants and preschoolers will outgrow their fatness. Interfering may distort their natural growth and development. But if the child is still overweight by age 11, and especially during adolescence, it's more likely to persist long term.

In a University of Iowa study, over half of children and teens from the highest of five weight categories remained in this same category as adults. On the other hand, nearly one-third dropped down into the lower three quintiles.[32]

The following age data compiled by Leonard Epstein, PhD, from four studies, shows the likelihood of obesity tracking into adulthood:[33]

Age of obese child	Percent who become obese adults	Relative risk
0-6 months	14%	2.3
6 months - 5.5 years	20	3.4
7 years	41	3.7
10-12 years	70	6.0

The relative risk of the overweight child becoming an overweight adult increases with age.

Epstein says this indicates when interventions might be helpful.

It also suggests the importance of not overreacting. About 60 percent who are obese even at age 7 will not be obese as adults.

Obesity that starts in adolescence tends to be more severe than adult-onset obesity, and most adults with severe obesity were overweight as adolescents, says obesity specialist William Dietz. He notes this is especially true for women: about one-third of all adult obesity in women began in adolescence; and obesity is less likely to change for women than men.[34]

CHAPTER 7

Lifestyle choices
increase problems

■

The problem of unhealthy eating goes far beyond the dinner table. So do the problems of a sedentary lifestyle. How children learn to eat and the activity habits they develop now can affect them the rest of their lives. Even stress has its effect on weight and eating problems.

In Canada, kids and adults are encouraged to enjoy eating well, to be active and to feel good about themselves, clearly the best way to prevent weight and eating problems.

But we in the United States don't get that message. And the results are disturbing, even shocking. After many years of teaching children and families about healthy living, I was appalled, but hardly surprised, by recent reports that many American girls are severely undernourished.

The startling truth is that most teenage girls do not eat enough for health, energy and strength. They are discouraged from competing in sports. And they feel so bad about themselves that one-third report having seriously considered suicide in the past 12 months — double the rates of boys their age.

What is the problem? Why are so many girls disheartened? Why are so many malnourished and undernourished, starving in the midst of plenty?

Restricting food

The answers to these questions, I believe, are in a culture that encourages girls to restrict their eating in unhealthy ways. There's also been a decided change in the kinds of foods young people eat.

A recent national study showed the median intake for girls ages 12 to 19 — what the girl in the middle is eating — is only 51 to 67 percent of the Recommended Dietary Allowance for calcium, iron, vitamin A, magnesium, zinc, copper and other critical nutrients. It's about 80 to 85 percent of recommended calories.

The RDA provides an allowance over minimum, yet these statistics mean that half of all girls are eating much less, and it's in this lower half where most of the deficiencies occur. Nutrients fuel growing brains and bones as well as strong bodies, but these girls aren't getting even the calories they need for healthy growth and development. They are severely undernourished.

Will these girls develop into well-rounded, capable, healthy adults? Or will they face a lifetime of health problems, like osteoporosis because they have kept vital nutrients from their bodies? Will they have financial troubles because they were too weak to learn in school and develop careers? I think the odds for future health problems are frightening.

The documentation for this appalling news is in the Third Report on Nutrition Monitoring, published by the U.S. Department of Health and Human Services and the U.S. Department of Agriculture at the end of 1995. It brings together information on nutrition from several surveys, analyses and monitoring systems.[1]

Unfortunately, even this report is missing the needed breakdown so nutritionists can see more than just medians and averages to evaluate what's going on. What's happening with the hungry one-fourth of girls at the bottom? This is what nutritionists need to know, but it's only available in a stack of unpublished pages at the National Center of Health Statistics. In these, the analyses are figured on one-day, 24-hour recall.

Adequate diets

Children start out eating healthy diets, but as they reach adolescence, their diets change. The Bogalusa Heart Study of children in the American South documents these trends. The number of kids eating only two-thirds or less of recommended nutrients increases for teens. The kinds of foods they eat also change toward more high-calorie, low-nutrient foods, more dessert and snack foods, more soft drinks.

It's puzzling that even though the children in the Bogalusa study are heavier than those studied 14 years ago, they eat fewer calories and less fat and cholesterol. Other studies show the same thing. But it's not clear if today's children are heavier because they are more sedentary or if somehow the dietary changes they've made may be causing new weight problems.[2]

The same trend is seen in other countries. A French study of 10-year-olds found that the children ate fewer calories, less total fat, and a lower percent of fat in 1995 than in 1978. Yet they had higher rates of obesity, 14 percent compared to 6 percent in 1978, and a more dangerous abdominal fat distribution. What's going on here? The researchers say this puts the origins of obesity into question.[3]

What are kids eating?

Young people today are eating twice as much as youth 15 or 20 years ago of foods like crackers, popcorn, pretzels and corn chips. More grain-based foods. More pasta with sauce, rice dishes, tacos, burritos — and pizza, the all time favorite. Three times as much soda pop. More desserts and candy.[4]

What's missing? They consume less meat, eggs and milk, and are still short on fruit and vegetables.

Half of teenagers drink no milk, compared with only one in four in the 1970s. Those who do, drink only about one and a half to two cups a day on average, not the recommended three to five glasses. Except for younger children, few eat the recommended five daily servings of fruits and vegetables.

The favorite vegetable is potatoes, often eaten as french fries and potato chips, followed by tomato dishes. Low on the list are green beans, corn, green peas, lima beans, and nutrient-packed dark green and deep-yellow vegetables.

Cave man diet

An odd thing about this kind of diet: It's almost directly opposite what our early ancestors ate. Prehistoric humans ate a high-meat diet with lots of fruits and vegetables. Food choices focused on these three food groups (after weaning from mother's milk at age 4 or 5). They ate almost no grain, according to anthropologists.

In Europe big-game hunters of 30,000 years ago were tall and strong with massive bones. They grew six inches taller than their descendents who settled down to farming, raised grains, vegetables and fruit, and seldom had animal products to eat. And it took their descendants until the Industrial Revolution, when they again ate more meat, eggs and milk, to gain back that height.[5]

Today, nutritionists advise that a sound food plan contains balance, moderation and variety from five food groups — grains, fruits, vegetables, meat group, and milk group. These fill the food pyramid. And at the top is a small niche for fats and sweets, special foods to eat sparingly (see Food Guide Pyramid in chapter 12).

Now we are seeing our children shifting diets away from modern advice for balancing the five food groups, and even farther from that ancient diet of three groups, to focusing mostly on a single group — a diet based largely on grains: bread, pasta, cereals, baked goods, crackers. Plus, youngsters today are pulling down those niche foods from the tip of the pyramid — desserts, candy, high-fat snacks, soft drinks — and expanding them into a major part of their diet.

This is a significant departure from five groups eaten in moderation, balance and variety — to focusing on one group, without much variety. It's extremely limited. How can it be healthy? Why are parents allowing it? Can it be because many parents are also eating this way?

Some parents think they can fill nutrition gaps with pills and supplements. But they are fooling themselves. Real food is what counts in a healthy diet, not supplements.

For example, take phytochemicals, one of the hottest new areas in cancer research. It's estimated there may be over 100 different phytochemicals in just one serving of vegetables. We haven't identified them all, much less which ones are most effective against cancer. Other nutrients and their roles are just beginning to be discovered.

This is why variety is so important in food choices, to ensure getting some of all needed nutrients. If you take a pill instead of real food, or instead of eating a balanced diet, you lose out.

Who's undernourished?

Teenage girls age 12 to 15 have the poorest diets of all Americans and are most at risk from nutrient deficiencies. They are followed closely by the older group of teenage girls, age 16 to 19. The report on nutrition monitoring shows that even at the median, most girls are deficient in many important nutrients.

By age 12, parents have less to say about what girls are eating, and nutrition may suffer. Girls this age are often into dieting, skipping meals and restricting foods. Yet they are going through puberty, which is an emotionally critical time for girls and a time when they need increased nutrition.

An adequate intake of calories and protein is essential for the growth and maintenance of a healthy skeleton, according to the Surgeon General's report on Nutrition and Health.[6]

In this early teen group, half of all girls have intakes below the median level and are consuming less than 57 percent of the iron and the calcium they need, in a one-day, 24-hour recall.

The hungry one-fourth

Much worse off are the teenage girls below the 25th percentile. For the most part these are hungry, even malnourished girls. When we look at the intake of the girl at the 25th and 10th percentile the severity of their nutrient deficiencies becomes clear.

For example, recommended daily calorie intake is 2,200 with a range of 1,500 to 3,000 calories for girls age 12 to 15. At the 10th percentile Mexican American girls are consuming only 833 calories, white girls, 904 and black girls, 1,064. At the 25th percentile level Mexican American girls are getting 1,300 calories, white girls, 1,358 and black girls, 1,400 calories. None of these girls is even up to the lower range of recommended daily intake for girls their age, set in

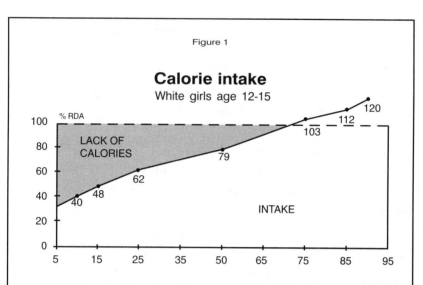

Figure 1

Calorie intake
White girls age 12-15

At the 25th percentile white girls consume 62% of their recommended daily calorie intake (RDA: 2,200). At the 15th they get 48% and at the 10th, 40%. Mexican American girls consume somewhat less, black girls somewhat more. One day 24-hour recall.[1]

UNPUBLISHED DATA, NHANES III, 1988-91/AFRAID TO EAT 1997

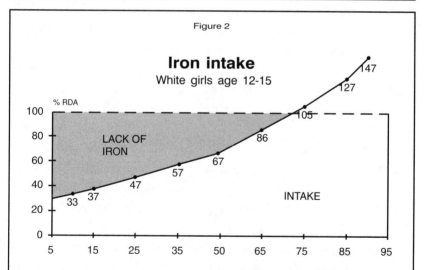

Figure 2

Iron intake
White girls age 12-15

Most teenage girls are deficient in iron. At the 50th percentile white girls are getting only 67% of recommended daily intake (RDA:15 mg); at the 25th percentile, 47%; at the 10th percentile, 33%. This means all girls below these points are getting less iron. Mexican American girls get somewhat less iron, black girls somewhat more. One day 24-hour recall.[2]

UNPUBLISHED DATA, NHANES III, 1988-91/AFRAID TO EAT 1997

1988 *(figure 1)*.

For iron, teenage girls at the 10th percentile are getting only one-third of the RDA, while at the 25th they are getting less than half of the iron they need *(figure 2)*.

The calcium situation is even worse. At the 10th percentile, girls are getting only 20 percent of the RDA requirements for calcium; at the 25th, slightly more than one-third *(figure 3)*. In fact, 87 percent of girls, ages 12 to 19, are not meeting the RDA — the amount of calcium considered essential to build a strong skeletal structure for a lifetime.

Even so, the RDA for calcium may be set too low. The American Academy of Pediatrics recommends increasing teen requirements from the milk group to five servings a day, rather than the three servings currently being recommended.

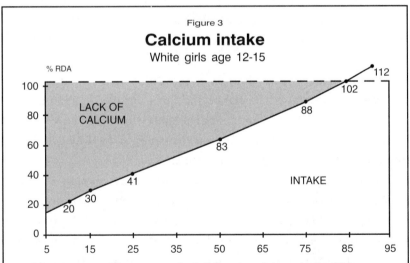

Figure 3

Calcium intake
White girls age 12-15

Most teenage girls are severely deficient in calcium. At the 50th percentile white girls are getting only 63% of recommended daily intake (RDA:1,200 mg); at the 25th percentile, 41%; at the 10th percentile, 20%. Mexican American and black girls get less calcium than this at the 25th percentile, more at the 10th. One day 24-hour recall.[3]

Unpublished Data, NHANES III, 1988-91/Afraid to Eat 1997

As can be expected, teenage girls are also extremely low in many other nutrients. At the 10th percentile they are getting barely half the protein needed, one third of the vitamin B_{12}, one-fourth of the zinc, and 15 percent of the vitamin A that is recommended.

Teenage boys, too, are generally low in calcium. At the 10th percentile they are getting only about 20 percent, and at the 25th one-third of the calcium needed.

It should be recognized that these percentiles are not averages, but the top intake for the lower 10 percent and the lower 25 percent of kids. Average intake for youngsters in the lower 10 percent or 25 percent would be much lower than this.

Deficiencies in iron and calcium

Two of the most critical nutrients for healthy growth and development are iron and calcium. Most teenage girls in the U.S. consume less than two-thirds of what they need.

Girls especially need iron because they lose iron-rich blood every month after puberty. Iron carries oxygen through the blood to cells, helping to produce energy. Girls who are low in iron will likely feel fatigued, weak, listless, irritable and have headaches. And they'll have a harder time learning.

The damage young children suffer from lack of iron may be irreversible. Mental performance fails to improve in treatment for many anemic children, some studies show. Iron-deficient children commonly have shortened attention spans, lower intelligence scores, and reduced overall intellectual performance.[7]

Iron isn't easily absorbed by the body. In fact, experts say up to 90 percent of iron consumed is lost unless some heme iron from animal products is included. Even a small amount of heme iron from meat, poultry, fish or eggs helps the body absorb iron, so vegetarians need to plan carefully to compensate. Vitamin C also aids in iron absorption.

Calcium is important for every child to maximize bone development, but it is even more critical for girls. They're building bone mass until about age 25. Girls who don't drink enough milk, and especially if they are thin and often dieting, may be setting themselves up for a lifetime of fragile bones, fractures and osteoporosis. Osteoporosis (literally, "porous bones") is painful and expensive. Women with severe cases can break their ribs sneezing, or break a leg or a hip by standing the wrong way. It can rob women of an independent and active life.

Experts fear an epidemic of osteoporosis when today's thin, dieting teenagers reach mid-life.

Perhaps if these girls would help out in nursing homes or visit the unfortunate women crumpled down into themselves, whose skeletons are giving way, maybe they'd value the strong bones they could be building now.

Why don't they drink milk? They fear milk is fattening. Why don't they eat iron-rich meat and eggs? It's the same sad story. Their fear of fat. (Even though they could eat these foods with very little or no fat).

Iron and calcium are only two of several dozen nutrients often deficient in poor and unbalanced diets like we are seeing in this "hungry one-fourth" of teenage girls. These deficiencies can cause long-term or even permanent health problems related to growth and development and mental problems such as depression, confusion, hysteria and psychosis.

Preteen girls

Overall, girls age 6 to 11 have more adequate nutrition. Yet even in this group, at the 25th percentile, white girls are getting only about half the calories recommended. This is set at 2,400 calories with a range of 1,650 to 3,300, somewhat higher than older girls because of special growth needs at this age.

Even though their RDAs for calcium are set lower than for older girls and these younger girls usually drink milk, many have diets low in calcium. At the 10th percentile white girls in this preteen group are getting 46 percent of needs; at the 25th, 69 percent.

Children are many different sizes and builds at this age, and their growth spurts will differ widely, so it is difficult to determine reasonable RDAs. Usually the RDAs carry an extra allowance. Yet the low calorie and calcium intake of the lower quarter of girls is a big concern.

Apathy in the press

After more than two years, and six years after data gathering ended in 1991 for this first phase of NHANES III, these statistics still have not been completely analyzed or published.

I keep urging that a clearer analysis be made of girls' food intakes and some action taken to reduce deficiencies. But health policy makers brush it aside, saying, "The big concern now is obesity, so we need to look at weight problems first — it's the priority." The figures are available only by special request from the National Center for Health Statistics.

It's true obesity is an urgent concern; many youngsters are overeating and eating too much of high-fat foods, and this needs to be analyzed as well. But it seems to me starvation is even more urgent; some youngsters are dying of malnutrition, and others may be dying from suicide related to starvation-induced depression. They are not dying from obesity.

Yet when the nutrient report with median intake levels came out in October 1994, it did not even hit the national press. Many experts are still unaware it exists. Even while listing only median levels this report should be cause for concern about girls, although it's not as alarming as a closer inspection of intake for the lower one-fourth. Now the data is collected for the second phase (1991-1994) but only calorie intakes are being analyzed at this time, and again concern focuses at the higher end.

In both the media and public health bureaucracy, there appears to be an overwhelming apathy toward the plight of adolescent girls. The attitude seems to be that dieting and losing weight is normal for girls, so deficiencies are expected. Any blip in obesity rates merits headlines worldwide, but malnourished girls get only a shrug and silence.

"We have become all too familiar with sociocultural studies supporting the fact that young women in our country are badly in need of attention, that they are being cheated, invalidated, and robbed of their voices," charges Paula Levine, PhD, an eating disorder specialist in Miami.[8]

Missing out on meat

That children and adolescents are missing out on meat is a serious matter that needs to be addressed by pediatricians, nutritionists and health policy makers.

It has become trendy and politically correct in the media and certain health circles to denigrate the contribution of meat to the American diet and to call for low-meat diets. This is not supported by mainstream nutrition. There is no credible evidence that eating lean red meat is unhealthy in any way, and volumes of scientific evidence that show meat is health-promoting, especially for children, teens and women. But this trendy notion is having a profound impact on the health and growth of children in America today.

Certainly vegetarianism can be healthy, but as being practiced by young people today, often it is not. We need to respect children's decisions on food choices, yet this can be a serious health issue. When youngsters choose to give up meat, there is concern about how they are doing it and to what extremes they might go.

From coast to coast, eating disorder specialists tell me they are seeing many new young vegetarians — small children with eating problems, stunted growth, fragile bones, and stress fractures, who are responding to a frightening message brought by animal rights activists into their schools. They also see a second kind of new vegetarian — eating disordered girls who fear meat is fattening.

"This is very dangerous for kids," says William Jarvis, PhD, Loma Linda University, president of the National Council Against Health Fraud.

Jarvis says ideologic vegetarian extremism has caused mental and growth retardation in children, is linked to nutritional rickets and scurvy, and in some cases, the deaths of children. They suffer the digestive distress that is common for vegetarians.

After many years of living and teaching in a Seventh-day Adventist academic community and having been a practicing vegetarian himself, Jarvis questions the motivation of the new young vegetarians. "As a religion, vegetarianism attracts the guilt-ridden. It attracts masochists because it gives guilt a boost. And it seduces the unskeptical by causing guilt and/or by instilling false guilt. Guilt leads to self-denial, even asceticism . . . Vegetarianism is riddled with delusional thinking from which even scientists and medical professionals are not immune."[9]

Today, many impressionable children and teens are being influenced by this kind of delusional thinking.

Two radical fringe groups are exerting tremendous pressure on children, teens and college students to stop eating all animal products. They are the overzealous environmentalists who mistakenly believe all land can be cropped and that grazing livestock wastes land, and radical animal rights groups determined to convert young people to the vegan lifestyle while abolishing pets, zoos, research and farm animals, and use of leather and silk clothing.

These groups have been extremely successful in manipulating the media. In denouncing animal rights tactics, the American Medical Association says, "The AMA continues to marvel at how effectively a fringe organization of questionable repute continues to hoodwink the media."[10]

Theirs is a dangerous agenda that calls for investigation.

Patricia Hunt, a registered nurse in Mukilteo, Wash., whose daughter Jennifer became a vegan after an animal rights group came into her school, recently told the *Wall Street Journal* she was "angry with the schools and the propaganda."

Hunt says Jennifer refuses even to take vitamins prescribed by her doctor because they are made from animal products. "She has a hotline number that she calls before she'll take anything."

Parents from Maine to California complained in the *Journal* article about animal rights activists and the teachers who invited them into the classroom to push the vegan lifestyle. No longer able to influence their children's healthy eating, these parents were further frustrated in being harangued by their kids about cooking ingredients, compelled to fix two sets of meals, and lectured about their own eating.

"There is a sense that these kids have been traumatized . . . influenced by the message that the animal rights people are taking into the schools. When children see these gory pictures about mistreated animals, they really don't have the ability to stop and say

'Wait a minute, is there another side to this story?'" explains Monika Woolsey, MS, RD, a nutrition consultant and eating disorders specialist in Arizona.

Woolsey has noticed a trend in her practice in which young adolescents often give up meat soon after having watched a graphic movie about meat processing by animal rightists. "These films may be inappropriate for children who are not equipped to handle the trauma they may inflict."[11]

She says vegetarianism seems to be a politically correct way to have an eating disorder. "Many of these children have suffered from emotional, physical or sexual abuse or trauma, and it's almost as if they've made a vow not to hurt animals as they have been hurt."

They struggle with self worth, says Woolsey. "They believe their self-esteem comes from what they do, not who they are, and part of what they do is eat. So they are trying to eat perfectly, and they get this black and white sense of what is perfect: 'If I'm a nice person I'll be a vegetarian, and if I'm not a nice person I'll eat meat.' That's how black and white their thinking gets when you talk to them."

In Kentucky, dietitians have launched an educational campaign to inform educators and parents about the threat of animal rights misinformation and deception being targeted to their schools.

Nancy Tullis, RD, chair of the Reliable Nutrition Information section of the Louisville Dietetic Association, says, "Self appointed 'nutritionists' should not be allowed to go into the schools to present an emotional diatribe about society's shortcomings in the areas of nutrition, air, soil, water and animal cruelty, place blame on certain groups, and then irresponsibly teach the new vegan diet pattern, leaving some inadequate brochures behind. The children will go home short on facts and long on anger. We do not believe in setting children up for this emotional confrontation with their families." *(See Appendix C for more information on this issue.)*

Cutting fat

In the past decade, both children and adults have reduced fat from an average 36 to 34 percent of total calories, bringing them closer to the goal of 30 percent or less fat set by the Dietary Guidelines for Americans.

High fat intake is known to contribute to obesity, and is a risk factor for chronic disease.

All things being equal, calories from fat (chips, crackers, candy bars, pizza, ice cream, margarine, butter, mayo) are stored as body fat much more easily than other calories. Fat is easily converted to body fat, unlike carbohydrate of which one-fourth of the calories are used up in conversion, and protein, for which little if any is stored as fat. Before discovering this and its link to chronic disease, Americans were eating an average of 41 to 42 percent of their total calories in fat — plus 25 percent in sugars. This left only about one-third of calories for other, more nutritious foods.

There have been positive changes in reducing fat intake — but the new awareness has led to a deep fear of fat.

Fear of fat

Some young people have taken their fear of fat to the extreme, developing fat phobias and reducing their fat intake dangerously low. A downside of the informative food labels is that they make it easier for fat phobic people to plan diets with "zero" fat.

This is painfully apparent in working with young women on college campuses. Cynthia DeTota, MA, RD, University Nutritionist at Syracuse University in New York, tells me that college girls' obsession with thinness and dieting is excruciating. Fat has become an evil.

At one sorority, girls who ate food containing any fat during rush week were required to pay into a penalty pot. In a drama group, students told her the newest trend is if a food has any fat "you can eat, but don't swallow. Spit it out!"

Girls in campus cafeterias typically choose a meal of only a lettuce salad with nonfat dressing and a Diet Coke. Many have taken up smoking to control weight.

"It's such a frustrating problem, because when I start talking about the dangers of over-restricting fat, these young women don't seem to value their health enough to make any changes. The value they place on physical appearance and body weight outweighs the value they place on their health," says DeTota.

"I have analyzed some students' fat intakes to be only four percent of their needs. When I give them the results, they are proud instead of concerned. They have an intense fear of fat. They really think if they increase their fat intake, they'll immediately gain weight.

"I encourage them to try a small change just for a week, anything else is overwhelming: 'If you could add one or two tablespoons of peanut butter on your bagels at breakfast. Just try it for a week and see if it makes a difference in how you feel.' Some will do it, and they say they feel so much better, are more alert, and don't fall asleep in class. But many are afraid to try."

Teenage girls who are eating in the recommended range of about 2,000 calories, balanced with physical activity, can maintain their weight and meet the recommended 30 percent fat with about 600 calories in fat, or 67 grams. This means averaging a comfortable 22 grams of fat at each of three meals. It's a long way from zero fat.

Another result of the current fear of fat is that many popular lowfat foods substitute double or triple the sugar for fat.

Some professionals are debating whether dropping fat down to 30 percent of the diet may be too low for children.

Lowfat diets are not appropriate for children or the elderly, insists Alfred Harper, PhD, professor emeritus of biochemistry at the University of Wisconsin. Harper faults the U.S. Dietary Guidelines because they are being applied to children. "These guidelines represent a sharp change in direction in health policy and dietary guidance, away from dietary advice to ensure that growth and development of children will not be impaired — and toward a program of dietetic medicine to prevent chronic and degenerative diseases," he told attendees at the 1996 Southern California Food Industry Conference in Costa Mesa, Calif.

Harper said the assumption that limiting fat intake in children will provide them with healthier lives as adults has not been validated by research.

He also questions why the current drop in fat has not been accompanied by a decrease in overweight, as expected, but rather by a sharp increase. While others suggest this stems from reduced activity, Harper argues that lowfat foods may be making people fatter because they lose the satiety cues formerly relied on. Perhaps they do not feel as satisfied with the foods they are eating today, often processed and prepackaged, as when eating home-cooked foods in family meals at home, he says.

Harper also argues that blaming fat for the increase in chronic disease is a myth. The increase in these diseases is a natural consequence of a healthier aging population that has overcome acute infectious diseases with improved medicine, he points out. Most people no longer die young. They die in old age of chronic disease — and that's as it should be, he suggests.

Skipping breakfast

Dieting teens commonly skip breakfast and thus miss out on a nutritious start for the day. So do many parents.

Recent reviews of the research confirm that starting the day without breakfast affects thinking, problem solving, verbal fluency, attention span, educational achievement, and ability to recall and use newly acquired information. Breakfast is especially needed by youngsters who are nutritionally at risk, or are dieting, one study shows. Iron deficiencies, anemia, and other nutrition deficiencies found to be prevalent in these youth severely affect their thinking ability.

Children ages 9 to 11 who eat breakfast are faster and more accurate in school and have better memories in these studies. Schools that provide breakfast find kids are more likely to come to school and they perform better in the classroom.[12]

Kids are also eating more food outside the home, which probably contributes to their often unbalanced food choices. One-third of students get nearly half their calories away from home, up considerably from the 1970s. Teenage boys report eating more often at fast food restaurants than at the school cafeteria.[13]

Confusing the public

Often family lifestyle choices make the difference between whether children develop weight and eating problems or not. Key factors in healthy food choices are moderation, balance and variety in mealtime eating. We need to return to these principles.

But it seems that Americans often go to extremes instead of choosing a moderate course. We're impatient. We feel like we're not making important changes unless they're *big* changes. If fat tastes good, overeat; if it adds pounds, opt for *zero* fat. On the one hand people feel sensuously indulged, on the other, austerely virtuous.

Can we forgo this drama of all or nothing mentality? Can we find peace with food and let this misplaced excitement flow into other interests?

The media eggs us on. One of the biggest barriers to reasonable food choices at this time is the confusion in the media over foods and health. Parents are fearful over the many supposed risks they read about daily in newspaper headlines. Children reflect this confusion and fear.

The problem is, in this time of instant communication, we get an overload of unimportant information. Newspapers cannot resist featuring the health terror message of the day. Scare headlines warn of the risks of white bread, popcorn, peanuts, Mexican or Chinese food, mad cow disease or alar treated apples. The public gets this startling news, and while it is here today, gone tomorrow, people are left shaken, a bit more fearful.

On a recent flight from Chicago, where I was a guest on the Oprah show, I sat next to a Kentucky businessman who traveled often.

"I was on a plane when the morning headlines in *USA Today* read, 'Coffee raises cholesterol,'" he told me. "No one drank coffee. On another flight the headlines said coffee might prevent suicide, and everyone was calling for coffee. Another time it was orange juice, and everyone drank orange juice. We're crazy, aren't we?"

Right. And headlines sell papers. Nevertheless, the media needs to be more responsible in helping people put these bits of information into perspective.

Some sources quoted may be barely credible. Others appear to be irresponsible, headline-grabbing researchers. They get lots of press. Experts today are often embarrassed and chagrined by "health terrorist" messages beamed out by researchers who should know better.

Two who have done more than their share of this lately are a group that calls itself the Center for Science in the Public Interest, which stayed a million hands in mid-reach for movie popcorn and devastated Chinese takeouts for a time, and the so-called "Harvard group," with its never-ending, sometimes-inappropriately reported Nurses' Study. (Why don't these scientists use well-sampled national databases to test their theories?)

The paradox is that this national panic over food and health comes at a time when Americans are healthier and living longer than ever before, and when the U.S. food supply is the best it's ever been, and without doubt one of the safest and healthiest in the world.

In actual fact, many of the headlined risks are negligible. If they made any difference at all, it might be only three or four days of longevity for a few individuals. Studies may be very preliminary, or represent one unorthodox view of an obscure controversy. Often the reports are meant for scientists talking to scientists, better discussed in a college lab than the front page of the daily newspaper. Also, headline seekers and groups with a political agenda have learned to manipulate the media to their ends.

And some of this fearmongering about food may be a deliberate smoke screen laid over smoking issues, according to Elizabeth Whelan, president of the American Council on Science and Health. She claims the nearly $6 billion spent yearly by the tobacco industry on advertising and promotion, plus the deep roots the tobacco industry has forged throughout corporate America, and the financial support it gives members of Congress "clearly buys silence and diversion" to hide the fact that half of all premature deaths before age 80, a half million each year, are directly and causally related to tobacco. She says nothing could make "this killer advertiser more content than having the word 'carcinogen' used so often it loses all its meaning. Remember: when everything is dangerous, then nothing is. The leading cause of death has enough clout to keep the legislative and publicity spotlights off the cigarette — and on the multitude of nonrisks around us."[14]

Instead of hearing clear messages promoting health, what we get is scare-mongering, an endless parade of "good foods" versus "bad foods," negativism and contradictions.

Harper regrets the trend toward categorizing foods as either good or bad, as medicines to heal us or health hazards that will shorten our lives. It's important to restore confidence in the basic principle that health depends on the total diet, not on a few special components. "This is of particular concern with the diets of children," he says.

Measures of despair

Eating well and living in healthy ways contributes to feeling good about ourselves. But if suicidal thoughts and plans are an indication of how our youngsters are faring, they are not doing well. Girls especially are in trouble.

Nearly one-fourth of high school students nationwide reported they had seriously considered attempting suicide during the 12 months before the 1995 Youth Risk Behavior survey, a slight increase over 1993 *(figure 4)*.

The rates are twice as high for girls, and highest of all for Mexican American girls. Of these Mexican American girls, 34 percent reported seriously considering suicide, 26 percent made a suicide

Figure 4

Suicide thoughts and behavior
percent of high school students

	Thought seriously about attempting suicide	Made a suicide plan	Attempted suicide one or more times
Female	30%	21%	12%
Male	18	14	6

Suicide-related thoughts and behavior of U.S. high school students during 12 months preceding the survey, as self-reported.[4]

1995 YOUTH RISK BEHAVIOR SURVEY/ AFRAID TO EAT 1997

plan, 21 percent attempted suicide, and 7 percent made a suicide attempt that required medical attention, all during the past year. For white girls these figures are 32 percent who considered suicide, 22, 10 and 3 percent, respectively; for black girls, 22 percent who considered suicide, 16, 11 and 4 percent, respectively.

For white boys the suicide behavior rates are: 19 percent reported seriously considering suicide, 15 percent made a suicide plan, 5 percent attempted suicide, and 2 percent made a suicide attempt that required medical attention. For black high school boys, the corresponding statistics are 17, 13, 7 and 3; for Mexican American boys, 16, 13, 6 and 3 percent.

Youngsters in the U.S. are twice as likely to commit suicide as in other developed countries. The rate is 55 in 10 million children, compared with 27 for the rest of the industrialized world. Suicide rates quadrupled among U.S. children under age 15 between 1950 and 1993, according to the Centers for Disease Control and Prevention.[15]

In the Behavior study, girls were more likely to have considered, planned or attempted suicide when they were younger, as freshmen or sophomores than seniors. This trend was somewhat reversed for boys. What's going on with these girls? What part might malnutrition-induced low moods and depression play? What about their struggle with body image and low self-esteem? Does sexual abuse play a role? What's happening to Mexican American girls to cause such despair? We need answers to these questions to bring about healthy change.

Physical activity

Young children are the most active and physically fit of all Americans, averaging one to two hours of moderate or vigorous physical activity each day. But they're less active than their parents were as children — and they're developing habits that could turn them into inactive, unhealthy, overweight adults.

Most grow less active each year. Many girls, in particular, drop into sedentary lifestyles by age 15 or 16. Others, when they stay vigorously active, focus only on their desire to lose weight or prevent weight gain. They see this as the sole reason to exercise.

Researchers find a relationship between the widespread decrease in physical activity and the increasing prevalence of obesity, even though it's difficult to measure both physical activity and its relation to obesity in children.

What is clear, is that both children and adults live less active lives than their peers a few decades ago.

Many families have changed their lifestyles in response to violence or feelings that they're unsafe in their communities. More parents work longer hours. More conveniences and remote controls save us the effort of getting up to switch channels or open the garage door. There are more TV channels, more computer games, video movies to watch, and hours of Internet to surf. And the 21st century only promises more, not less, of these kinds of sedentary recreation.

Below recommended levels

The 1996 Surgeon General's report on Physical Activity and Health finds over one-third of high school students are not active at recommended levels (20 minutes or more of vigorous physical activity for which you have to "sweat or breathe hard" at least three days a week). One-fourth don't engage in any vigorous activity at all.

Boys are more active than girls, and the gap widens through high school and college, says researcher James Sallis, PhD, of San Diego State University. He found that both boys and girls (like adults) think they are more active than they really are.

Girls may be at higher risk of activity-related health problems due to their more sedentary lifestyles, warns Sallis.

Yet the outlook has improved greatly in the last decade. Schools are doing a better job and more youngsters are more active. The major concern is the lower one-third. We're close to meeting the Healthy People 2000 objective in which 75 percent of children ages 6 to 17 will exercise vigorously 20 minutes at least three days a week.

The Surgeon General's report uses several large national studies, including the Youth Risk Behavior survey of high school students, and the National Health Interview survey of young people age 12 through 21. In the Behavior study nearly two-thirds of high school students are active at the recommended level. This includes about three-fourths of boys and half of girls (74 vs 52 percent). For boys, these statistics are 76 percent of white, 70 percent of Mexican American, and 68 percent of black students. For girls, the figures are 57 percent of white, 45 percent of Mexican American, and 41 percent of black students who are sufficiently active.

The study looking at ages 12 to 21 reports somewhat lower activity. About half of U.S. young people this age are active at recommended levels. The percentages are double the 1990 figures, but represent a slight drop from 1993.

Students with higher income tend to be more active, and all kids are more active in the spring than any other time of year.

Decline in activity with age

Physical activity of all types declines strikingly as kids get older *(figure 5)*. Girls show a steep drop from their freshman year to senior year — from 61 percent who are active as freshmen to 41 percent as seniors. However, this drop was even more severe in 1990, when fewer girls were active and it fell from 31 percent to 17 percent by senior year.

Boys show a similar decline from 81 percent as freshmen to 67 percent as seniors. The study looking at older youth found by age 21, activity had dropped further to only 42 percent for boys and 30 percent for girls.

Inactivity is defined as performing no vigorous activity and no light to moderate activity (walking or biking for 30 minutes) during any of the seven days before the survey.

For the age group 12 to 21, the National Health Interview Survey shows inactivity is higher for girls than boys (15 percent vs 12 percent), and increases with age. Overall, for boys, there was little difference among racial and ethnic groups.

In the high school survey fewer kids were inactive (14 percent of girls and 7 percent of boys), suggesting that after they get out of high school there is a further drop in activity. However, slightly more black girls (21 percent) were inactive in the high school study. This compared with 12 percent of white girls and 15 percent of Mexican American girls.

Lifetime skills in PE class

The reputation of physical education class was never stellar. Despite many recent improvements, research shows that in many classes, students still spend more time standing in line or watching others perform than being active themselves.

One study found that a 40-minute physical education class provided youngsters with an average of less than three minutes of vigorous activity.[16]

"It appears that a major opportunity to influence favorable physical activity in the United States is being missed in schools," says one Public Health report. The report points out that physical education

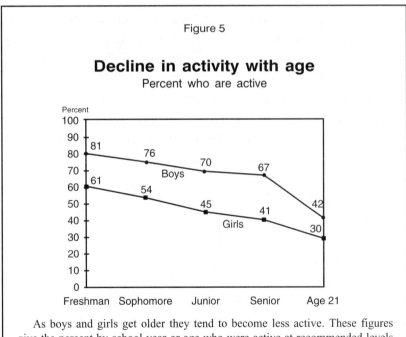

Figure 5

Decline in activity with age
Percent who are active

As boys and girls get older they tend to become less active. These figures give the percent by school year or age who were active at recommended levels in the 1995 NHIS-YRBS surveys and Surgeon General's Report on Physical Activity.[5]

NHIS-YRBS, 1991-1995/Afraid to Eat 1997

classes seem to have little effect on the students' fitness levels or on increasing their lifelong physical activity.[17]

Despite their criticisms of how physical education is often taught, most researchers urge higher enrollments in daily PE classes at all age levels.

Sixty percent of high school students are enrolled in PE classes, but only about one quarter attend classes daily, a decline from 42 percent during the first half of the 1990s. Healthy People 2000 aims to increase this to at least 75 percent. In an average PE class, 70 percent of the students spend at least 20 minutes exercising — about half a typical class period.

Nonathletic and less fit youngsters, the other 30 percent, are the ones who need PE the most. Yet they are most neglected. One in six U.S. children is so weak or uncoordinated as to be considered physically underdeveloped by the President's Council on Physical Fitness and Sports.

"That cold statistic barely hints at the personal trauma and social problems behind it. Such a child is likely to become a sedentary, overweight adult with all of the added health risks those conditions entail," says the Council.

Most schools still emphasize competitive sports, ball-handling skills, winning games, and showcase the best athletes. It's a system with little but humiliation to offer the unathletic or overweight child.

It's time to focus more effort on identifying and helping physically underdeveloped children, says the President's Council. This is "the most urgent task facing physical education and other youth activity programs."

Girls, and especially black girls, urgently need attention from athletic directors.

The Council urges schools to test for fitness, as they do for reading and math, and enact remedial programs for students who don't meet standards. A special class is recommended, or if this is impractical, a separate exercise program for part of the session or the entire class participating in activities needed by the underdeveloped.

Most of these kids can achieve appropriate levels of physical fitness, say experts. Teachers and parents need to understand the importance of fitness for each child in healthy growth, academic performance and prevention of weight problems.[18]

Physical education classes are further criticized for what they teach. Games and competitive sports, rather than lifetime activities, are the major focus of most existing programs. Federal researchers point out that for physical education classes to contribute to the health goal of lifelong activity, they should include moderate-intensity activities and should not focus exclusively on team-oriented sports activities.

The 1985 Children and Youth Fitness Study found that less than half of the PE curriculum was based on lifetime activities. These are activities that require only one or two people and are readily carried into adulthood, such as bicycling, swimming, jogging, dancing and racquet sports. Competitive sports and children's group games do not count as lifetime activities.[19]

Kinds of activity

Half of all students play on at least one school sports team, with girls almost as likely to play on school teams as boys (42 vs 58 percent). But boys are much more likely to play on sports teams outside of school — 46 percent compared with 27 percent of girls.

About half of high school students do strengthening and toning activities at least three days a week. Boys are more likely to do these than girls, and white students more than black students. And again, freshman girls are more likely to do them than older girls.

Walking or biking for 30 minutes at least five days a week is used as a measure of light to moderate physical activity. This declined from 26 percent of high school kids to 21 percent between 1992 and 1995. Black and Mexican American students, both boys and girls, are more likely than white students to have walked or bicycled. Light to moderate physical activity decreases with age and is more prevalent in fall than other seasons.

Seven additional types of activity were surveyed in the Fitness study: aerobics or dancing; baseball, softball or frisbee; basketball, football, or soccer; housecleaning or yard work for 30 minutes; running, jogging, or swimming; skating, skiing, or skateboarding; tennis, racquetball, or squash. Boys are more likely to participate in these activities, except that girls are more likely to engage in aerobics, dancing, house cleaning and yard work. All decline as they get older, except for cleaning and yard work.

Nearly two-thirds of girls said the reason they exercised in the month before the survey was to lose or maintain weight. So did one-third of the boys.

Girls discouraged from sports

Girls have many more opportunities and participate more in sports than ever before, yet experts say they have a long way to go before they are treated equally.

Sallis says the evidence suggests we need to reevaluate the reasons girls are less fit than boys. It has been thought that fitness differences are related to girls' lower muscle mass, higher body fat and hemoglobin concentrations as they mature. But maybe that's not the major reason. Maybe this new data suggests that the continuous decline in girls' aerobic power is the result of their declining activity. Sallis urges this be explored further and warns that girls need more effective programs to prevent this decrease.

Girls are still neglected in physical education. Often their enthusiasm is actively dampened by family, friends, the institutions in charge of sports and health, and by what they see in the media. They get far less encouragement in sports than boys.

Historically, women's sports were thriving during the 1920s and 1930s, and most high schools fielded girls' basketball teams. But a changing national mood after the second world war ended this. Girls' teams were dropped in the late 1940s, as men returned from the war and "Rosie the Riveter" went back to her kitchen. In the ensuing "feminine mystique" era, vigorous sports were deemed too strenuous for girls. The mood in those post war years encouraged femininity and the protection of girls. According to prevailing belief, sports could harm the health and development of young women.

Iowa was one of the few states to continue girls' basketball through this period. Most states failed to reinstate girls' sports until required to do so in the late 1960s and early 1970s, when Title IX brought more equality for girls in high school athletics.

Yet most girls drop out of sports in their teens, and considerable evidence shows their self-esteem drops, too, at this same time.

Melpomene, a Minneapolis-based women's sports research organization, is asking why this happens and how girls can be helped to continue their interest in sports. A recent Melpomene study finds younger girls, age 9 to 12, enjoy sports and describe them as a way they feel good about themselves. But older girls, age 12 to 17, while agreeing that they enjoy sports, cite major obstacles. Among these are the behavior of boys and systems that favor male athletes.[20]

These girls said boys on mixed teems control the games. Typical comments:

"Boys, they like to hog the basketball."

"Even if you're right there, they won't pass the ball."

"In soccer we have half the girls standing out most of the time because all the boys are playing."

This male control was also evident in picking teams. The girls said boys were chosen first: "Girls are always last."

Some girls said they hesitate to play on these mixed teams for fear of male criticism or of making a mistake. The girls also described a system in which boys have more team choices, better equipment, and are taken more seriously by the school and fans.

"At boys' games the whole stands are filled . . . basically the parents are there (for girls)."

"They get better coaches, more time, more fields to play."

The researchers were concerned that in focus groups teenage girls commonly prefaced their remarks with "I don't know."

The girls often said this before giving an opinion or fact, such as, "I don't know, I just love sports."

They cite research that shows girls enter adolescence full of confidence and sure of what they know, but three years later are unsure of themselves, and their knowledge becomes private.

Using the qualifier "I don't know" was seen as a way the girls protected themselves from criticism. In one focus group this qualifier was used almost 50 times to preface the girls' opinions. More use seemed linked to lower self-esteem, confidence and competence, the researchers report.

News stories

Despite the encouraging example of the 1996 Olympics, girls have comparatively few female athletic role models. Media coverage often ignores women's teams and women athletes.

When the media does focus on women in sports, it is often in a conflicting and confusing way that sends mixed messages to young girls. Female athletes are frequently portrayed in ways that emphasize their femininity, rather than their athletic skill and excellence in their chosen sport. This can cause much ambivalence for girls, uncertain whether their role is primarily athletic or looking attractive and feminine on the field.

Amy Terhaar Woodcock, a graduate student in sports management at the University of Minnesota, says reporters watch for female weaknesses and then often exploit them in photos and stories. She explains that the media has tried to find a way for female athletes to continue to fit into our culture's feminine ideals by pointing out that women are too frail for contact sports.

She cites references which document how the media focuses on "sex specific rather than sport specific conditions or injuries" for women but not men. An injury which to a male athlete is attributed to the sport, is for a female athlete blamed on female weakness.

Sports magazines such as *Sports Illustrated,* avidly read each week by sports-minded girls and women as well as men, typically devote more space to swimsuit editions, pinup calendars and cheerleaders than to women athletes.

One study of *Sports Illustrated* covers from 1957 to 1989 found a decline in the number of times women were featured in active poses over these 22 years. Men were featured on the cover 782 times, and women 55 times. But of these 55 covers, only two showed women in active poses.

Another study examined pictures of female Olympic athletes and found the photos were often suggestive, emotional, or the women were shown away from their sport. Many focused on the female athlete's body in sexually suggestive ways. Emotional shots showed the athlete crying and being comforted by male coaches and family. Most of the photo captions mentioned feminine characteristics and often that the woman was short, rather than pointing out her athletic skill and achievements.

Women's sports are vastly under-represented in television, newspaper and sports magazines. A look at four daily newspapers found that women were the subjects of only 3.5 percent of all sports articles, and men, 81 percent. Men were pictured in 92 percent of all sports. Another study showed men's professional golf was shown 70 times on national television in 1993, while women's golf appeared only 13 times.

Woodcock studied the daily newspaper coverage of girls' and boys' high school ice hockey in the Twin Cities area in 1994-1995.

She found there were 65 boys teams and 24 girls teams in the Metropolitan area, but 89 percent of the newspaper space was devoted to boys' hockey, compared with 11 percent for girls' hockey. Articles on boys which had photos averaged 43 inches of print. Articles on girls with photos averaged 11 inches. The boys' stories had an average of one more photo per story and they were often action shots. Of 35 photos of girls' high school hockey, only four showed the girls actually playing hockey.

When a female hockey player was chosen athlete of the week, she was pictured sitting on a bench holding her stick and gloves. An article headlined, "Small Stature, Big Talent," showed a photo that emphasized the girl's small size by cutting off her teammates' heads. The article referred to her as the "tournament darling." In a more positive portrayal, another newspaper featured the same athlete by focusing on her athletic talent, mentioning her size once, and running a photo that showed her on the ice, in uniform, shooting a puck.

This unequal newspaper, television and sports magazine coverage is reflected in sports books — even picture books for very young children.

A Melpomene Institute study found that even today girls are portrayed only about half as often as boys in picture books on sports which are aimed at children under grade two. Often girls are shown watching boys in action.

These are major improvements, however. During the 1950s and 1960s, no girls at all were shown in this sample of books. The researchers looked at 105 books from the last 40 years containing 23 popular sports sampled from the sports category of the children's picture book directory *A to Zoo.*

Overall, nearly three times as many sports books from the last four decades had males as the only or major characters compared with females (58 percent to 20 percent). Males were identified as the only characters four times as often as females. Gender equality was portrayed in 17 percent of the books.[21]

CHAPTER 8

Struggling with weight loss

■

Most American teenage girls are trying to lose weight, no matter what they weigh. So are one quarter of teenage boys. Some are children as young as 7 or 8, often using hazardous methods. And one of two adults diet.[1]

These alarming statistics raise many questions. What is happening to these children as they restrict nutrients and continually yo-yo their weight up and down? What happens to their growth, their bones, their brain development, their lives? Is this supposed to be normal? Are we going to accept it as normal?

Being overweight may have health risks, but that does not mean weight loss lessens those risks. Often it does the opposite. Losing weight and attempts to lose weight can be dangerous — potential risks include permanent injury and death. At the very least, the efforts they make to reshape their bodies are diverting many children from their important tasks of emotional and intellectual growth.

Who's striving to lose weight?

Who is trying to lose weight, struggling to become less than they are? Almost everyone. Several recent surveys show similarly frightening results: Most girls and a large percent of boys are dieting and trying to lose weight.

The 1995 Youth Risk Behavior survey found that during the last 30 days before the survey over half of white high school girls had dieted to lose weight or keep from gaining, along with half of Mexican American and one-third of African American girls.[2]

A nationwide Centers for Disease Control study reported that of 8th and 10th graders, 61 percent of girls and 28 percent of boys had been on a diet to lose weight during the previous year.[3]

Still another study of Cleveland teens found that 70 percent of white girls and 60 percent of black girls had lost at least five pounds in a weight loss attempt, as had 40 percent of all boys. More than one-third of these girls were currently dieting, including 40 percent of white girls and 38 percent of black girls. Many used dangerous weight loss methods, including semi-starvation, vomiting, diet pills, laxatives, diuretics and smoking. One-third of dieting girls and one-fourth of dieting boys said they fast for 24 hours at least once a week *(figure 1)*.[4]

"This is very disturbing," said Laurie Humphries, PhD, director of the Eating Disorders Clinic, University of Kentucky. "Frequently, we find these adolescents come in, 5-foot-1 and 100 pounds . . . and (say) they need to be 89 pounds."

"Our study confirms that high school students feel very pressured to shape their bodies into the popular mold, and that increasing percentages of both boys and girls are dieting and purging in an attempt to accomplish this," said Lillian Emmons, PhD, RD, the nutritional anthropologist at Cleveland State University who directed the study.

The high dieting rates she found among boys are much higher than earlier reports, and yet may be underreported, says Emmons. Of particular concern, she suggests, are the 10 percent of male dieters who lost 62 pounds or more through dieting, and lost 10 pounds twice as often as any other group.

Emmons says meaningful education on the dangers of dieting, and reasonable expectations for body size and shape, need to be taught in schools before the preadolescent growth spurt.

But this is not happening, or if it is, "is not as powerful as other cultural pressures. The amount of purging shown in this study is cause for concern because of the potentially damaging effects purging can have on health," she warns.

As noted earlier, not only are more kids dieting today, but they are starting younger. A California study found up to 81 percent of 10-year-old girls are restricting eating because of their fear of fat.[5]

Young athletes in sports and performance arts that emphasize leanness are at special risk for harmful attempts to control the size and shape of their bodies. These include gymnastics, wrestling, judo, boxing, weight lifting, bodybuilding, figure skating, diving, ballet, dance, horse racing and distance running.[6] Vomiting and laxatives are commonly used by female college athletes in several sports.[7] Many high school wrestlers use extreme fluid and food deprivation in their efforts to "make weight" for a match.

Figure 1

Dieting and purging
Percent of high school students

	Girls		Boys	
	White	Black	White	Black
Dieting	77%	61%	42%	41%
Liquid diet	14	24	6	9
Diet pills	23	16	6	0
Laxatives	7	18	5	2
Diuretics	5	11	1	2
Vomiting	16	3	7	0
Monthly or more often	8	1	–	–
Fasting monthly or more often	35	40	29	25

Potentially harmful dieting behaviors are widely practiced by U.S. high school students. Total 1,269 students, Cleveland State University study.[1]

HWJ/Obesity & Health Nov/Dec 1992/JADA 1992
Afraid to Eat 1997

A "hundred ways' to lose weight

Losing weight can be so difficult — and so profitable — that a huge industry has grown up around it. There are a hundred ways and more to lose weight, and children succumb to all of them, from diets, drugs, gadgets, smoking and purging to surgery — methods which can damage the body, mind and pocketbook. None of them work in a safe and lasting way for very many people, but each time they are led on to a new miracle "guaranteed" to work this time, again and again. The trick is that they seem to work for a time, so people keep coming back for more, seeking to discover their own "failure."

Dieting — in all its forms — is big business, with a price tag of $30 to $50 billion annually in the U.S. alone. The thinness culture has created a desperation in people from childhood to old age and profiteers are quick to move into the void.

Even the Food and Drug Administration is vulnerable to industry pressure. In April 1996 it approved a diet drug, dexfenfluramine (Redux), which had not been studied successfully in patients for more than one year. Yet to be effective the drug needs to be taken long term, perhaps for life.

These many methods are being used on and by children. They are combined and delivered in a variety of ways. Some are self-prescribed. Some are directed by lay leaders or counselors of varying competency, through clubs, support groups, commercial diet centers and summer camps. Still others are medically monitored in hospital settings by multi-disciplinary medical teams. Some are inexpensive; others cost thousands of dollars. Most often, the consumer, who may be a young child, quietly picks her own diets and diet products.

Some treatments are conservative, recommending a gradual weight loss of a pound a week or so. Others are radical, severe, and cause large, rapid weight loss and just as rapid rebound.

Treatment programs for large children and adolescents traditionally have emphasized food restraint and control. In the last 15 years most have added an exercise and behavioral component.

Weight loss methods being used today include:

- Dieting, restricting food
- Drugs

- Surgery
- Gadgetry, wraps, panaceas
- Exercise
- Combinations

Dieting, restricting food

Ways of restricting food include flexible or rigid diets, fasting, "detoxifying" the body and vomiting to eject consumed food before it can be digested. A diet limits calories and/or fat. It can specify certain foods or food combinations, or replace meals with liquid diet products. Low and moderately low calorie diets provide about 1,000 to 1,500 calories daily; very low calorie diets, 300 to 800 calories.

Very low calorie diets

Semi-starvation or very low calorie diets of under 800 calories have special appeal because you lose weight fast. Moreover, you lose appetite for awhile, so you don't even feel hungry. Expected weight loss is 22 pounds or more in 10 weeks.

However, lost weight is regained rapidly.

And risks are high. Even under medical supervision, very low calorie diets carry serious health risks, and these escalate steeply when kids engage in do-it-yourself fasting, fad diets and liquid diets at this level.

This kind of diet has the highest risk for sudden death syndrome, warn researchers at the National Institutes of Health Obesity Research Center in New York. Sudden death can come without warning or follow cardiac arrhythmias when the heart muscle itself loses size during large, rapid weight loss.

It also increases gallbladder disease risk. Children rarely develop gallstones, but one 13-year-old girl had to have her gallbladder removed after losing weight through a diet prescribed by the Doctors Quick Weight Loss Center. The girl was given a cursory physical plus a test for food allergies before beginning the program. Then she was given a list of foods she could and couldn't eat, supposedly based on the allergy tests, her mother, Loretta Pameijer told a congressional subcommittee that held hearings on the weight loss industry in 1990.

Although her daughter followed the diet faithfully, there were times when she would stop losing weight, Pameijer said. "The counselors would put her on a parsley break. It had almost nothing in it but meat and a half a cup of parsley a day."

The girl's physician said she had "the worst gallbladder attack" he had ever seen in anyone so young.

"We're angry because it never occurred to us to be suspicious of a doctors' clinic," Pameijer said.

A New York City investigation also turned up numerous injuries, including the case of a 15-year-old Long Island girl who had to have her gallbladder removed after losing 72 pounds in six months.

University of Alabama nutrition researchers find new gallstones in 10 to 26 percent of persons on very low calorie diets, some within the first four weeks.[8]

While there is much less support for very low calorie diets today amid the wreckage of their late-1980s heyday (when talk show host Oprah Winfrey publicly lost and regained weight on a liquid diet), many authorities still promote them. Regretfully, the prestigious 1995 book, *Weighing the Options*, by the Food and Nutrition Board of the Institute of Medicine, recommends very low calorie diets and other dieting for large children.[9]

"Dieting remains the cornerstone of therapy for the obese child," advises *Options*. It goes on to suggest liquid diets of 600 to 800 calories, with part of the calories made up by two to four cups of low-starch vegetables for kids. This is called a "protein-sparing modified fast," a somewhat outdated term, now being revived. (It was once claimed this would cause fat loss while sparing "protein" or muscle, but this was proved false.)

Options recommends this diet be reserved for high-risk kids, the "more serious cases of childhood and adolescent obesity, for which rapid weight reduction is essential."

Yet, it seems no child is too young: "In children, the protein-sparing modified fast has been used on children as young as 6 and by children whose weight ranges from 120 percent to greater than 200 percent of ideal . . . (However) in England, (it) is not recommended for children under 13."

It isn't explained why large, rapid weight loss can be considered "essential" or healthy for "the more serious cases."

Vomiting

One in six white girls in the Cleveland study vomit in a desperate effort to avoid digesting the food they eat.[10]

Vomiting can cause sore throat, difficulty in swallowing, heartburn-like pain, esophageal rupture, tooth decay, loss of potassium, dehydration and cardiac arrhythmias.[11]

Forceful vomiting may tear the mucosa of the gastrointestinal tract, revealed as blood in the vomitus. Occasionally, the force of vomiting can break small blood vessels in the eyes and injure the esophageal sphincter, allowing stomach contents into the lower esophagus. The esophagus can rupture after ingestion of a large meal and subsequent forceful vomiting. This is a medical emergency with very severe upper abdominal pain, worsened by swallowing and breathing. It has high death rate if left untreated; surgery is usually needed.

Low levels of potassium, essential for muscle and heart functioning, can trigger cardiac arrhythmias, from prolonged vomiting.

Some kids use Ipecac syrup to induce vomiting. Large doses are extremely dangerous and can cause cardiovascular, gastrointestinal and neuromuscular toxicity.[12]

Those who vomit three times a week or more will eventually cause erosion of their tooth enamel from acid vomitus in the mouth. Experts say this erosion can take as little as six months, or several years. Teeth get sensitive to heat and cold, develop spaces between, lose fillings, and eventually deteriorate down to painful cores.

Vomiting also causes "chipmunk" cheeks, probably from repeated gland stimulation by the acid contents of the stomach.

Dieting shrinks a woman's world

Dieting and fasting — even without nutrient deficiencies — can harm a child's mental and physical growth and development.

"Dieting is not just about eating, it is an entire way of life," warns Janet Polivy, PhD, a University of Toronto professor who has researched the detrimental effects of dieting for over 20 years. "Life has a different meaning for people when they become dieters. Their self-image and self-esteem is all tied up in this."

Polivy says the dangers of dieting include emotional and psychological harm, eating disorders, financial cost and diminished lifestyle. Her research shows dieters respond differently than non-dieters in a range of situations.

Chronic dieters are easily upset, emotional, have mood swings, are more likely to eat when anxious, and have trouble concentrating on the task at hand if there is any kind of distraction, Polivy reports. They are compliant and have a need for perfection, are preoccupied with weight and body dissatisfaction, have lost touch with internal signals of hunger and satiety and rely on cognitive cues for eating. They salivate more when faced with attractive food, and have higher levels of digestive hormones and elevated levels of free fatty acids in their blood. They can go longer without food and eat less under "ideal" circumstances than nondieters, but once started, they binge or eat more, then experience guilt.

A chronic dieter focuses on food, eating and weight, both for herself and in her perception of others, has lower self respect, is eager to please and compliant with the demands of others.[13]

Ellyn Satter says dieting causes a child to cross the line to external restriction of food, leaving behind natural weight regulation and normal responses to internal cues of hunger and satiety.

This is a profound change in eating and has serious consequences. The child learns to distrust his or her own responses and relies instead on external factors such as calorie count, food selection patterns, lists of dos and don'ts, and body weight.

And even so, the internal processes will not be ignored, she warns. "You have to invest more and more time and effort in overcoming the physical and emotional symptoms of energy deficit: hunger, increased appetite, fatigue, lethargy, irritability and depression. And you become preoccupied with food and with yourself. In some cases, these negative feelings become very strong, perhaps because the person is depriving herself terribly . . . and she just keeps trying harder and harder."[14]

Eating disorder specialists Linda Smolak and Michael Levine agree: "Although weight/shape concerns and dieting behavior are common in elementary school children . . . they are not harmless. In the short run, caloric-restrictive diets generate irritability, distractibility, food preoccupation and fatigue. The long-term effects are more worrisome. Dieting children may be at special risk for developing severe eating disorders . . . Caloric restriction during childhood and adolescence can lead to stunted growth, menstrual dysfunction and decreased bone density."[15]

One chronic dieter says dieting made her less of a human being. "What I resent about dieting is that it makes one so terribly self-centered, so much aware of oneself and one's body, so preoccupied with things that apply to oneself only, that there is scarcely any energy left to be really spontaneous, relaxed and outgoing. It starts with thinking about what to eat and what not to eat, and gradually goes over to other fields, and it is this aspect that makes me resent dieting; it makes me less of a human being."[16]

"Dieting shrinks a woman's world," says Merryl Bear, coordinator of the National Eating Disorder Information Centre in Toronto.[17]

Dieting is abnormal

The problem with dieting is that we are not able to integrate diet behavior into our normal lifestyle because it is abnormal, says Mary Evans Young, founder of No Diet Day and author of *Diet Breaking*.[18] "Dieting is based on deprivation, sacrifice and guilt, which are difficult to sustain. We lose touch with our natural hunger signals in responding to external cues which don't address underlying issues."

Diets wreck lives, undermine health, sap confidence, self respect and energy. Dieting affects nearly all girls and women, diverting them from facing their real issues, preventing many from fulfilling their potential, and causing obsession with food, body and weight.

The diet industry has the perfect product, Evans Young observes. "It promises so much, and when it doesn't deliver the consumer blames herself and then goes on to the next diet." Yet dieting can make girls feel they are doing the right thing. They feel good just for having made the decision to go on a diet. Pursuing thinness is widely

Risks of dieting and weight loss

Mental and emotional risks

- Apathy
- Depression, anxiety
- Irritability, intolerance, moodiness
- Decrease in mental alertness, comprehension, and concentration
- Thoughts focused on eating, weight and hunger
- Self-absorbed, self-focused, decrease in wider interests
- Preoccupation with own body, judgmental of others' size
- Lowered self-esteem, feels self-worth depends on being thin

Physical risks

- Weakness, fainting, fatigue
- Cold intolerance
- Gallstones
- Gouty arthritis
- Cardiac disorders
- Elevated cholesterol
- Anemia
- Headache
- Elevated uric acid levels
- Loss of lean tissue
- Nausea
- Diarrhea, constipation
- Edema
- Hair loss and thinning hair
- Hypotension
- Abdominal pain
- Muscle cramps
- Aching muscles
- Both slowed and increased heart rate
- Heart abnormalities, arrhythmias
- Death[2]

HEALTH RISKS OF WEIGHT LOSS, 1995/AFRAID TO EAT 1997

perceived to be the same as pursuing good health.

"That feeling of self-sacrifice can hook us into wonderful feelings of purity and goodness," notes Evans Young. "The diet becomes a kind of fanatical religion, requiring you to abide by a set of stringent rules or pay the penance of guilt. It's a guilt that starts by slowly nibbling and then steadily gnaws away at your body, spirit and confidence. Give yourself a break. You deserve much, much more."

Drugs for weight loss

Drugs used for losing weight include prescription drugs, over-the-counter diet pills, fraudulent pills, laxatives, diuretics, herbal weight loss tea, gum, appetite sprays and nicotine (smoking). Claims often made are that the drugs will reduce appetite, increase metabolism, block digestion, and/or "flush out fat" stored in the body. Most of these are illegal claims.

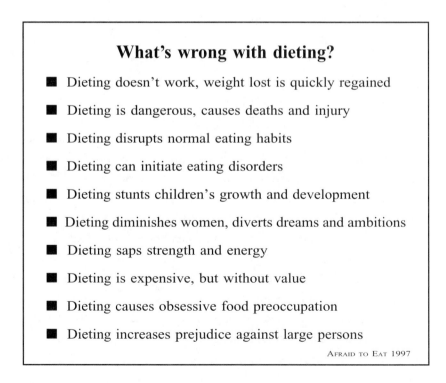

What's wrong with dieting?

■ Dieting doesn't work, weight lost is quickly regained

■ Dieting is dangerous, causes deaths and injury

■ Dieting disrupts normal eating habits

■ Dieting can initiate eating disorders

■ Dieting stunts children's growth and development

■ Dieting diminishes women, diverts dreams and ambitions

■ Dieting saps strength and energy

■ Dieting is expensive, but without value

■ Dieting causes obsessive food preoccupation

■ Dieting increases prejudice against large persons

AFRAID TO EAT 1997

The new diet drugs

The new prescription diet drugs — fen/phen and Redux — are flying off pharmacy shelves all across the country as advertisers promote and people demand and many physicians eagerly prescribe.

Yet, the truth is these new diet pills don't work very well and can be extremely dangerous. We recently reviewed the research in *Healthy Weight Journal* and found that over the course of one year these drugs increase weight loss by an average of only five and a half pounds over taking a placebo or "sugar pill." Most weight loss apparently comes not from the pills, but from the prescribed diet. It's the same old story, in which people lose weight quickly, then regain it all, except for those five and a half pounds — which stay off as long as the pills are taken.

It's hard to believe that people will continue taking this costly pill just to keep off less than six pounds.[19]

And these drugs are dangerous. They've been determined safe for only one year by FDA, but are being prescribed for long-term and even "lifetime" use.

One of the most serious side effects is primary pulmonary hypertension, a disease that's fatal within four years for nearly half those who get it. Either drug could cause an estimated one case per year for every 22,000 to 44,000 patients who take the drug longer than three months. (And there's no point in taking it a shorter time, as the weight is regained upon stopping the pills.)

Brain damage is also documented in more than 80 animal studies. Evidence of brain disturbances in humans show up in sleep disturbances, depression, and psychotic reactions. In addition, a long list of potentially severe reactions are listed on the Redux package insert (as required) and should not be taken lightly.[20]

Even health policy makers and the usual promoters acknowledge these pills can be harmful. The National Task Force on the Prevention and Treatment of Obesity recently advised, "Until more data is available, drug therapy cannot be recommended for routine use in obese individuals, although it may be helpful in carefully selected patients." The Task Force also advised against giving these drugs to children and adolescents, except in clinical trials.[21]

Yes, sometime in the future we will have targeted weight loss drugs that are safe and effective for most people. But not yet. And our vulnerable children have time to wait.

PPA pills off the shelf

You don't need a prescription for diet pills off the shelf. Many teenage girls confess they shoplift and swallow the pills by the box.

Pills containing PPA (phenylpropanolamine) are readily available everywhere at grocery, drug, chain and convenience stores, under such names as Dexatrim, Accutrim, Control, Dex-A-Diet, Diadex and Prolamine. PPA is the only over-the-counter weight loss drug approved by the FDA, except for benzocaine which is seldom used (said to numb the tongue).

Parents and health professionals have pleaded with FDA and Congress to restrict PPA diet pills to prescription sales for adults.

A bereaved father at the 1990 congressional hearings protested their easy availability. "The lights went out in our lives on July 12, 1989, when our beautiful, fun-loving, and soon-to-be-married daughter, Noelle, died of cardiac arrest. These stores have no more business selling these drugs to children than they do liquor to a minor."[22]

Vivian Meehan, president of the National Association of Anorexia Nervosa and Associated Disorders, urged Congress to require that diet pills, laxatives, diuretics and emetics be sold to adults from behind the counter, never from an open shelf or near products identified as diet aids, and to minors only by prescription.

Approved as a diet aid in 1979 (when it was believed effective), PPA has been placed "on review" by FDA, a move that can sidetrack action for years. Over $40 million dollars is spent annually on advertising the profitable PPA diet products.

One in three teen girls has taken diet pills in some studies. In the Cleveland study, white kids used them more often than black kids, up to 23 percent of white girls, compared to 16 percent of black girls.[23]

In a survey of Michigan State University students, one in five said they'd started using PPA diet pills between age 12 and 16. Nearly half the women and 6 percent of the men had taken a PPA dietary drug. About 27 percent of the women had taken it within the past 12 months and 3 percent in the past 24 hours.

None had ever consulted a physician, even though labels advise it under age 18. Many took more than the recommended daily limit of 75 mg of PPA. About one-fourth of the women students using diet pills had also double-dosed, using other PPA-containing products at the same time. PPA is also found in cold medicines and one young woman with a severe cold had taken a diet pill and four nonprescription decongestant products containing PPA within 24 hours of the interview — a total of 675 mg.

Diet pills may cause a rebound effect of fatigue and hyperphagia, insomnia, mood changes, irritability and, in extremely large doses, psychosis, say Allan Kaplan and Paul Garfinkel in *Medical issues and the Eating Disorders.*[24] Other documented side effects include fatal strokes, dangerously high blood pressure, heart rhythm abnormalities, heart and kidney damage, hallucinations, seizures, headaches, nervousness, cerebral hemorrhage, nausea, vomiting, anxiety, palpitations, renal failure, disorientation and death.

Even when used correctly, PPA can cause dangerous reactions. It leads all other major nonprescription drugs in the number of adverse drug reactions and in the number of contacts with Poison Control Centers, a total of nearly 47,000 in 1989.

Furthermore, most users say PPA doesn't work in weight loss, and no data at all contradicts this.

Quack pills and potions

In addition to PPA pills are the many quack pills, illegally claiming that they suppress appetite, speed up metabolism, block digestion of fat or calories, flush fat out of the cells, or otherwise alter body functions to bring about "safe, easy, fast" weight loss. Often sold as "natural" or "herbal," these products are usually labelled as food supplements to avoid being confiscated by FDA. The claims you saw in the ad or the TV infomercial are nowhere to be seen on the label.

Pills like these are often singled out for the Slim Chance Awards we give each January from *Healthy Weight Journal* and the National Council Against Health Fraud, for which I serve as national coordinator of the Task Force on Weight Loss Abuse. Awards go to the four or five "worst" weight loss products of the year. Always in hot competition are the latest versions of "all naturals," bee pollen, chromium picolinate and herbal pills.[25]

Ephedrine, often sold as the Chinese herb Ma huang, or for legal purposes as an asthma remedy, has proven one of the most deadly of the quack pills. In March 1994, 10 Texas teenagers were taken to emergency rooms after overdosing on ephedrine. After 37 hospitalizations and two suspected deaths, Texas Health Commissioner David Smith temporarily banned Formula One, a popular diet supplement containing ephedrine, and prohibited the sale of ephedrine products to young people under age 18.[26]

FDA warned consumers not to buy or ingest Nature's Nutrition Formula One products that contain both Ma huang (ephedrine) and kola nut. Overdosing with ephedrine can start the heart racing, cause heart palpations and death. Yet overdosing is common with diet pills. In the past two years, the FDA reported over 800 adverse reactions to ephedrine-containing products including at least 17 deaths. Reactions included life-threatening conditions: irregular heartbeat, heart attack, angina, stroke, seizures, hepatitis and psychosis. Temporary conditions such as dizziness, headache, memory loss, and gastrointestinal distress were also reported.[27]

Bee pollen, too, has caused fatal allergic reactions. FDA warns that bee pollen holds hazards for anyone with allergies, asthma or hay fever — although promoters claim it is "naturally safe" and "safe for any dieter."[28] Authorities in Australia recently linked royal bee jelly to a severe asthma attack that killed an 11-year-old girl.[29]

Weight loss fraud works because people want to believe there are easy ways to lose weight. Con artists exploit this with a mixture of mysticism, pseudoscience and sensationalism, says Burton Love, FDA Midwest Regional Director. Authorities say there is more fraudulent and misleading information about nutrition and weight today than ever before, and it is being marketed more effectively in high-tech, highly targeted ways, with enormous profits.

There's an endless supply of these "magical" quack pills for weight loss, endlessly hyped. In the last 12 years I've reported on hundreds of questionable diet products in *Healthy Weight Journal* and our special report *Weight Loss Quackery and Fads,* and have stacks of advertisements on these kinds of products awaiting review. If these ads find me, they're finding the kids, too.[30]

Amphetamines

Amphetamines are no longer recommended because of potential addiction risk, but are still available and being prescribed by some doctors. In their youth, many of today's large people were prescribed amphetamines and struggled with addictions.

Gloria, now 43, was prescribed her first diet pills at age 12. In the book *Real Women Don't Diet,* she explains, "They weren't called 'yellow jackets' or 'uppers' back then. They were just some little yellow pills given to a physically healthy 12-year-old to lose weight . . . Withdrawing from years of diet pills, which meant having vivid hallucinations and periods of extreme paranoia and finally becoming bulimic, were the most dangerous, physically damaging aspects of my war with my body, but the psychological damage and pain have been far more lasting."[31]

Marcia G. Hutchinson, now a psychologist and author of *Trans-forming Body Image,* recounts similar experiences. "From a very early age, I was subjected to state-of-the-art diet methods — amphetamines at age 6, a 10-day hospitalized water fast at 15, and a dizzying array of restrictive regimes in between."[32]

Laxatives and diuretics

Taking laxatives or diuretics is a dangerous and ineffective way to lose weight. In the Cleveland study African American girls were most likely to use laxatives and diuretics — 18 percent had used laxatives and 11 percent diuretics in attempts to lose weight. About half of users took these pills at least every month.[33] In the 1995 Youth Risk Behavior Survey, laxatives and diuretics were more common among Mexican American and white high school girls than black girls, (11, 8 and 4 percent, respectively).[34]

Laxatives cause weight loss through dehydration due to a large volume of watery diarrhea. Calorie absorption is not really affected but nutrients may be poorly absorbed.

Abuse can cause both acute and chronic lower gastrointestinal complications, including abdominal cramping, bloating, pain, nausea, constipation and diarrhea, says the National Eating Disorders Organization.[35] Laxatives can result in the loss of electrolytes, including potassium, essential for heart function.[36] Chronic abuse may cause nerve damage resulting in sluggish bowel that can get so severe it requires removal of the colon, replaced by a colectomy.

Tolerance develops to laxatives over time, so abusers may increase to 60 or more tablets daily. Laxatives are probably the most common type of drug abused by bulimic patients.[37]

Diuretics or "water pills" are used less by youngsters, but their abuse is extremely dangerous. The big concern is potassium loss leading to heart arrhythmias and kidney damage. Using several purging techniques together intensifies the effects. A physician should be consulted immediately on signs of potassium loss, such as muscle weakness, fatigue and chest pain.

Herbal tea

Herbal weight loss teas cause fatalities, too, warns the FDA.

Of particular concern were reports to FDA of at least four recent deaths in women who drank Laci Le Beau Super Dieter's Tea. All died suddenly, and three of the four had cardiac effects. All used the tea several times a week.

Similar teas the FDA looked at were Trim-Maxx, 24-Hour Diet Tea, and Ultra Slim Tea. Adverse effects from these teas ranged from diarrhea, cramps, fainting and permanent loss of bowel function, to death. Many teas for weight loss contain large doses of stimulant laxatives such as senna, cascara, castor oil, buckthorn, aloe and rhubarb root. These are used in over-the-counter laxatives — but in smaller, well-controlled dosages.

Since the teas are sold as food supplements, they're not regulated and contain unknown amounts of laxative. Potency varies widely with growing season, amount used, and steeping time.

Smoking to lose weight

Nicotine is probably the most "successful" weight loss drug, the most common and one of the most hazardous being used today. And smoking rates are up for young people, especially girls. White high school girls now for the first time ever are smoking more than boys. There's one compelling reason: to control their weight *(figure 2)*.

One in three high school students smoke occasionally (at least one cigarette a month), according to the 1995 Youth Risk Behavior survey. This is highest for white students at 38 percent, with 34 percent for Mexican American and 19 percent for black students. White girls have even higher rates at 40 percent, compared with 37 percent for white boys, and 12 percent for black girls.[38]

White girls are also most likely to be frequent smokers (20 cigarettes or more a month). Twenty-one percent smoke frequently, compared with 18 percent of white boys. Rates for Mexican American students are about half those of whites; for black males much lower and for black females, only 1 percent.

Smoking has its own powerful industry promoting nicotine as a method of weight control. I've been looking at ads in magazines read mainly by girls and women and find they almost invariably use the word "slim," usually in a subliminal way such as "slim price."

The jump in girls' smoking began during his tenure in the late 1970s, "to the point where for almost two decades teenage girls have been puffing away at rates exceeding or equal to those of teenage boys," mourns Joseph Califano, Jr., former secretary of Health, Education and Welfare. He says he regrets not dealing with the fear of weight gain early in the fight against smoking.

Targeting women in cigarette advertising began in the late 1960s, he says, and in the next 20 years death rates from lung cancer increased 500 percent for female smokers.[39] And girls and women are not as likely to quit as males.

With teenage girls leading the way, 3,000 American adolescents become regular smokers every day. "Virtually all will be sicker than the rest of the population, most will never quit, and more than a third face early death as a consequence of their addiction," says Califano. He says the nation's obsession with thinness is a great boon to tobacco companies and they play shrewdly on the fear of weight gain.

"That's what makes Virginia Slims and Capri Superslims —

with their names, slim cigarette outlines, and extremely thin models — so attractive to teenage girls."

Smoking is starting younger, according to a Healthy People 2000 report. Of high school students who have ever smoked, about one-quarter smoked their first cigarette by sixth grade, one-half by eighth grade, and three-fourths by ninth grade. It's harder to quit when kids start early, and they are more likely to become heavy smokers and develop a smoking-related disease, says this report.[40]

The tobacco industry denies targeting children, yet advertizes heavily in magazines kids read, sponsors sporting and concert events that attract young people and get wide television coverage. It favors the image-based ads most effective with youth, especially low-income youth.

Tobacco is responsible for more than one of every six deaths in

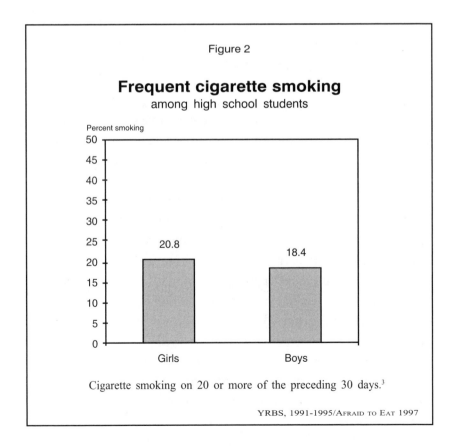

Figure 2

Frequent cigarette smoking
among high school students

Cigarette smoking on 20 or more of the preceding 30 days.[3]

YRBS, 1991-1995/AFRAID TO EAT 1997

the U.S., according to the Healthy People 2000 report. Smoking during pregnancy accounts for up to 30 percent of low birth weight babies and 10 percent of infant deaths.

However, numerous studies confirm the popular belief that smoking does help to keep weight down, and upon quitting smoking, most people gain some weight.[41] This effect is well-known to teens.

In national studies, smokers who quit gain an average of about 10 pounds above the weight gain of those who continue smoking, but their weight does not differ from that of persons who never smoked. This is consistent with other studies that show people who quit smoking "catch up" with their peers who don't smoke.

Thus, nicotine acts much like prescription diet drugs. Either way, people keep off five to 10 pounds and regain it quickly when they stop using the drug.

The Healthy People 2000 goal is to reduce smoking by youth so no more than 15 percent are regular cigarette smokers by age 20. But with the continued pressure to be thin by Healthy People 2000 itself and other entities, meeting this goal is quite impossible.

Surgery

Surgery for weight reduction can reduce stomach size, or shorten, alter or bypass various digestive processes. Other surgical procedures include liposuction, tummy tucks, jaw wiring and the stomach balloon (gastric bubble).

Surgery carries real risks and is not recommended for children under age 17, according to the 1991 Gastrointestinal Surgery Consensus Development Conference. Yet children are having surgery, and do die from it. A review of gastric weight reduction surgeries at the University of Florida Department of Surgery, Gainesville, showed three deaths within the first year among 11 children who had jejunoileal bypasses. Three others had severe complications requiring reanastomosis. Thirty-nine surgeries for weight loss were performed on adolescents from age 11 to 19 at that institution during the previous 11 years.[42] Nation wide, an estimated 15,000 people have weight-reduction surgeries each year. About 180, or 1.2 percent, are listed as being age 18 to 19.[43]

Death rate for this elective surgery is up to 2.5 percent in published studies, or five people out of 200 patients.[44]

Gadgetry, wraps, panaceas

In the quack arena are numerous acupressure devices, slimming earrings, appetite patches, passive exercise tables, electrical stimulators, slimming insoles, vacuum pants, battery-driven spot-reducing belts, body wraps, hypnotism, meditation, mystical panaceas, aroma therapy, Chinese slimming soap, spot reducing creams and lotions.[45]

Of the gadgetry and oddball methods, most involve con artists and quackery of one kind or another. It may be tempting to believe you can lose weight or build muscles by using a gadget or sticking a patch on your arm, but of course it doesn't work. The voice of the quack is seductive in enticing youngsters to spend money on items and promotions like these.

Exercise and its excesses

Being physically active is important in balancing what we eat, in maintaining health and our normal, healthy weight. We need to encourage physical activity and demonstrate how exercise fits into a balanced life.

Yet, at the same time, we need to be aware of exercise abuses, in which obsessive exercise can take over kids' lives and cause harm.

Obsessive exercising is closely linked to eating disorders, and has many of the same features. A key to when exercise becomes a problem is often when goals shift from enjoyment and becoming fit and healthy toward body reshaping. It is important for teachers and coaches to emphasize health-promoting goals, and question weight loss and muscle building. Girls may desire to fix what's "wrong" with their bodies. Boys are responding to a new emphasis on body sculpting and muscle building, conforming to advertising that is now teaching body dissatisfaction to males.

Karin Kratina, MA, RD, an exercise physiologist, dietitian and clinical outreach coordinator at the Renfrew Center in Florida, describes the typical scenario of a young woman with exercise dependence. "She rises each morning at 5:30, hits the pavement for a brisk

A doctor's weight loss education
by Allen King, MD

For the past 20 years I have seen over 5,000 obese patients for weight reduction and weight-related diseases. The results of my attempts to improve their disease state by weight loss were, at best, short-lived.

Initially, I thought obesity was caused by lack of knowledge. I gave patients an outline of the caloric content of foods. In a follow-up period of four weeks to four months, the average patient lost eight ounces. Half gained weight!

I next tried behavior modification and recruited a dietitian to provide a more individualized diet. In a three month follow up, the average patient lost only five pounds.

With the popular movement to liquid diets and their initial great success, I then tried a rigidly controlled program. Over 500 patients were placed on 500 to 1000 calorie diets with behavior modification. The average patient lost 50 pounds in six months. I felt we had finally succeeded. A three year follow up, however, uncovered an average 60 pound regain.

Certainly, I thought, what was needed was more control. Gastric surgeries were unacceptable due to the mortality and morbidity rate. Anorexic medications were of limited use. My two patients who elected jaw wiring lost weight initially, then regained. The Garren Gastric bubble seemed the ideal solution — a plastic balloon inflated in the stomach. Weight loss did occur, but only in patients who developed ulcers and bowel obstructions.

I then became disillusioned and found myself avoiding discussing diet approaches with patients. Each method was followed by failure, and worse, guilt on the patient's part for "failing."

I now realize it is not the doctor's role to control the patient. Responsibility for change is with the patient. Change takes time and progress is variable. I now tell patients it takes five years to change. Patients who are able to change benefit greatly from their increased self knowledge and self acceptance.[4]

Reprinted from Healthy Weight Journal. Allen King, MD, is currently using a nondiet approach in treating diabetic patients with Dana Armstrong, RD, in private practice in Salinas, Calif.

three miles, rain or shine, works out 45 minutes at the fitness center on lunch break, and goes to another health club after work for an hour of aerobics, half an hour on the Stairmaster and a half hour on the Lifecycle. She appears to be a motivated, fit and happy person but her legs ache constantly as she continues to work out, despite shin splints. When she stops for a time her depression and anxiety become so overwhelming, she can't wait to get back to her workouts."[46]

Kratina says at least half the anorexics and bulimics she sees probably deal with some form of exercise dependency. "Stress injuries are common, and frequently the person exercises right through an injury so it can't heal properly."

Amenorrhea and menstrual dysfunction are common for female athletes in many sports, often linked to weight restrictions. The "female-athlete triad" links eating disorders, amenorrhea and osteoporosis and is a known risk for elite women athletes.

Amenorrhea is associated with scoliosis and stress fractures in young ballet dancers. Delayed menarche, as late as age 19 or 20 for very thin female athletes and ballet dancers, usually with a restrictive diet, is linked to osteoporosis and bone fractures. (At the same time, a later puberty, well over the average age of 12.8, appears beneficial in reducing reproductive cancer risk.)[47]

Struggling to be best at a sport while coping with adolescent changes is difficult for girls because of social pressures promoting thinness. Trying to control weight while focusing on training and performance may lead to a sense of frustration, guilt, despair and failure, and to unhealthy eating and eating disorders.

Body fat dangerously low

The average young man, with normally about 14 to 16 percent body fat, will often strive for 5 to 7 percent if he is serious about sports in which leanness can be a factor, says the U.S. Olympic Committee's Division of Sport Medicine and Science. Girls, too, may try for extremely low body fat, even though they might normally have body fat of 20 to 22 percent. Measurements are notoriously inaccurate, so there's increased risk when body fat readings are low.

Severe dieting affects both the mind and body, but young athletes may not realize this. Garner and Rosen say young athletes may fear that the symptoms they experience — poor concentration, moodiness, irritability, anger, depression, feelings of inadequacy, anxiety, obsessional thinking, poor decision making and social withdrawal — are signs of deeper emotional disturbances.[48]

In calling for all states to raise body fat requirements for male wrestlers from 5 up to 7 percent, Charles Tipton, PhD, writing in the *Physician and Sports Medicine*, cites a study of elite high school wrestlers at the Iowa State Wrestling Championships which found 30 percent had only 5 percent fat or less.

There is overwhelming evidence, Tipton says, that calorie restriction will ultimately diminish muscle strength. While student wrestlers need 1,500 to 2,200 calories, he says, they often eat between zero and 500 calories on days before a match. The report says 7 percent of wrestlers use vomiting on a monthly basis, 1 to 3 percent have used diuretics or laxatives. One specialist in wrestling research warns that a sign of losing too much weight is loss of concentration and "a skinny kid walking around in a daze."

My two sons, Rick and Mike, both high school wrestlers in the lower weights, were dedicated wrestlers, champions many times, so I understand well the weight conflicts. Often I felt helpless in hoping for their good health despite their determination to "make weight."

The loss of three or four pounds is a big loss for the smaller 103-pound wrestler, compared with the same amount for a 180-pounder, but it is often treated as the same by the coach. The 5 to 7 percent error factor in even the best body fat measures is another problem, especially for the thin wrestler. More use of certified athletic trainers and nutritionists is being advised to minimize negative effects.

Making weight

A Pennsylvania study found 42 percent of high school wrestlers had lost 11 to 20 pounds at least once in their lives. One-fourth were losing 6 to 10 pounds every week. After a match, 30 to 40 percent reported being preoccupied with food and eating out of control. They used a variety of aggressive methods to lose weight, including dehydration, food restriction, fasting, vomiting, laxatives and diuretics. "Making weight" was associated with fatigue, anger and anxiety.

Weight loss methods were investigated with 42 college wrestlers by Suzanne Nelson Steen, MS, RD, and Shortie McKinney, PhD, RD. Most were reducing and depriving food and dehydrating. Over half had less than two-thirds RDA for vitamin A, vitamin B6, magnesium and zinc. One-fourth did not meet it for vitamin C, iron and thiamine. One-third ate less than recommended calories. This was more severe because RDA doesn't allow for their strenuous training. Diets tended to be higher in fat and lower in carbohydrate than recommended.[49]

Intake was extremely variable. One 118-pound wrestler ate 334 calories the day before the match, 4,214 calories in the evening after his match, and 5,235 the next day. His weekly loss was 12 pounds, followed by rebound after each match. Intake of food and fluid were typically minimal and sometimes zero for both days before a match.

Wrestlers consumed food and fluid in the five hours between weigh-in and match, but it was insufficient time to restore electrolyte balance or replenish muscle glycogen concentration. Many compete with greatly reduced carbohydrate stores, leading to premature fatigue and poor performance, the researchers found. On one team 5 percent of the wrestlers lost weight with laxatives and diuretics and 11 percent by vomiting.

"If there's a way to lose weight, a wrestler will find it," said Don Herrmann, associate director of the Wisconsin Interscholastic Athletic Association. "I've seen vomiting, laxative abuse . . . even a self-induced bloody nose."[50]

Among nutrition misconceptions was the common view that starchy foods are fattening. One-third avoided breads, pasta and potatoes. They reported cravings for sweets. After the season, wrestlers increased fat intake far above either preseason or midseason, suggesting that deprivation may have increased their preference for fat. Most ate well before and after the season.

Athletic trainers say rapid weight loss for wrestlers can cause kidney and heart strain, low blood volume, electrolyte imbalances, increased irritability, depression, inability to concentrate, and increased vulnerability to eating disorders. Severely restricting food and fluid can affect metabolism, body composition, performance, body temperature and overall health. Fluid losses and resulting electrolyte disturbances can increase risk of cardiac arrhythmias, renal damage, impaired performance and injury, say Garner and Rosen. Concerns are also raised about stunting during a period of active growth.

Most wrestlers used dehydration in the Steen and McKinney study. These included saunas (51 percent), wrestling in a heated room (74 percent), wearing rubber or plastic suits while exercising (42 percent), and restricting drinking (58 percent). Competing or training while dehydrated is an extremely hazardous practice. It inhibits sweating and increases risk of body temperature problems and heat stroke.

It's ironic, say Steen and McKinney, that 83 percent of the wrestlers correctly believed their sudden weight loss affected performance. They note that after a 4 percent loss of body weight from dehydration, muscle endurance drops 31 percent. Endurance was depressed as much as 21 percent even four hours after rehydration.

Bodysculpting

Weight training increases strength, endurance and bone density. It's a valuable part of high school athletic programs.

However, weight training and body building can become detrimental when youngsters' goals focus on reshaping their bodies for the sake of appearance. Coaches and trainers may also get caught up in muscle building, to the extent their influence can be harmful to youth. Athletic directors, coaches and parents need to be aware the new emphasis on muscle building and body sculpting is strongly influencing teenage boys through advertising, television shows and muscle magazines.

Joe McVoy, PhD, a Virginia eating disorders specialist, says he is seeing more boys with eating disorders who are overly caught up in bodybuilding. "This has become more epidemic because of the growth in our society of an emphasis on fitness and body shaping. There's a great increase in fitness and muscle magazines, fitness spas, and home exercise equipment all with a focus on shape and muscle building."

Bodybuilding competitions featured in muscle magazines are not about skill or strength. The emphasis is all on appearance, showing off the body. They're modelling contests for both men and women. Beyond having great muscle size and bulk, contestants deplete fat from under the skin, and dehydrate so severely that skin is thin as paper. This defines muscles, rope-like, and makes blood vessels stand out like veined leaves just under the skin's surface. Bodybuilders call this being "ripped" or "sliced."

This is competitive bodybuilding. The technique combines long hours of high-intensity training, extremely lowfat diet, depleting fluids in the final days before a contest, and for some, use of illegal steroids and prescription drugs. Steroid effects may be permanent and can put users at risk for heart disease and stroke. There are reports they may also increase aggressive behavior and violence. Dependency is another risk, according to Jim Wright, PhD, Health and Science editor of *Muscle & Fitness*.[51] He cites one study suggesting that at least one-fourth of high school users of steroids are dependent on the drugs.

Kids need education on the adverse effects of all of this. With the extreme efforts to reshape the body, abuses are common. Eating disorder specialists suggest that many young women are substituting bodybuilding for eating disorders, or combining the two.

Red flags for athletes

An obsession with a sport may be a "red flag" that an athlete is overtraining in unhealthy ways. Athletes at risk tend to talk and think about their sport constantly, often spending hours upon hours in the gym perfecting their workout at the expense of school activities, friendships and hobbies.[52]

Experts are calling for mandatory training for coaches to help them become more aware of obsessive exercise and eating disorders, and learn to watch for warning signs.

Nancy Thies Marshall, chair of the USA Gymnastics's task force on eating disorders and the youngest member of the 1972 US Olympic gymnastics team, has struggled with disordered eating. She offers these "red flags" for athletes, coaches and parents to watch for:

- Obsession with the sport. At the expense of family, friends, hobbies and school activities, the athlete at risk tends to devote herself to her sport.
- Preoccupation with food and weight. Thinking or talking often about food, fat and calories, frequent weighing, skipping meals and binge eating. Motivation for exercise may be a belief that losing weight will improve performance or appeal to a judge's eye.
- Drinking an overabundance of fluids in the effort to feel full.
- Laxative or diet pill use.
- Bathroom visits after meals. This may suggest the potentially fatal binge-purge cycle of vomiting food after eating.
- Wearing baggy clothing. Clothing may be used to hide weight loss.
- Dramatic weight loss.
- Physical deterioration. Malnutrition may cause chills, apathy, irritability, dry and pale skin, hair loss. Vomiting may cause callused finger, and sores on lips and tongue.
- Withdrawing from relationships. Feeling depressed, moody and lonely.
- Overexercising. Compulsive exercise beyond her regular workouts may be a sign the athlete is trying to compensate for eating.
- Menstrual dysfunction. Missing periods or delaying menarche for too long (perhaps beyond age 16 or 17) raises concerns of premature osteoporosis and bone fractures.[53]

Combinations

Weight loss programs often involve combinations of several methods, such as pills, diet and exercise. In the hope they will lose weight, many parents send their children to summer weight loss camps where various methods are used and combined.

But how good are these camps, and what do they have to offer? Perhaps not all that those concerned about children would like.

"Most camps are costly, stress excessive weight loss and fail to include an intensive family component," warns Laurel Mellin, RD, Director of the Center for Adolescent Obesity, San Francisco.

Mellin says that the typically severe dietary restrictions actually stimulate binge eating after camp is over. And since the family has not made changes to support a new lifestyle, the teenager's weight loss is unlikely to last long.

Such camps, Mellin points out, "are most likely to attract families that are desperate about their adolescent's weight and want to have their child fixed. The obese adolescent becomes the victim as parents first delight in initial weight loss, then despair and blame him or her as weight regain predictably occurs."

While some camping programs recognize the vulnerability of young people and hire qualified health professionals, many others do not. Some rely on staff with rigid views or lay staff who focus too much on exercise and restrictive diets. Young people at summer camps may be especially vulnerable to unfortunate weight loss experiences, Mellin suggests.[54]

A doctor in China seems to have taken the weight loss camp idea to the extreme. An Associated Press story tells of a 10-day weight loss camp for 60 children, ages 8 to 14, directed by Dr. Yan Chun, chief endocrinologist at Beijing Children's Hospital. Yan restricted his young campers to an 800 to 1,000 calorie, high protein, low starch, no-sweets diet. He exercised them four to five hours per day, and medicated them with a "new appetite suppressant." The program "seems to be working," the reporter wrote, because "the children's main topic of conversation was how much fat they'd shed."[55]

Industry gives 'guidance' to doctors

New guidelines for obesity treatment have recently been developed by the weight loss industry and two groups, the C. Everett Koop "Shape Up America!" program and the American Obesity Association. The *Guidance for Treatment of Adult Obesity* identifies six levels of weight and risk and calls for increasingly more aggressive intervention at each level. At the three highest levels it suggests drug treatment, very low calorie diets and, finally, surgery. As usual, it is not explained why high-risk patients should be subjected to high-risk methods. This might make some sense if the methods were effective. But there is no credible evidence of this.

The *Guidance* is distributed to physicians and will undoubtedly be regarded as an objective overview by many who are unaware of the industry influence. The *Guidance* is for adults, not children, but the suggested treatments likely will be used on youngsters.[56]

Laura Fraser, author of *Losing It: America's Obsession with Weight and the Industry that Feeds on It,* reports that former Surgeon General C. Everett Koop accepted $1 million each from Jenny Craig and Weight Watchers for his "Shape Up America!" campaign, which emphasizes the risks of obesity, suggests more Americans need to diet, and advises that companies and health insurance should pay for employees' weight loss programs. Koop was photographed with a smiling Jenny Craig in an 11-page advertising supplement in *Time* magazine. Nancy Glick of the Shape Up program admits that was a mistake and says they no longer allow Koop to have his photo taken with his commercial sponsors.[57]

I find it sad and ironic that a man long identified with the gallant fight against smoking should be part of an enterprise that puts so much pressure on girls to be thin, that they are turning to smoking as never before.

Failure of obesity treatment

Vast amounts of research money and effort are going into obesity treatment and its marketing. Yet, the fact remains: if even one of these hundred or more weight loss methods worked, would we have the others? I don't think so.

Take the example of polio. There were many "cures" and preventions for polio before one success ended it all — Salk vaccine. An entire industry was wiped out. Now there's no quackery left in polio.

While promoters continue to claim dramatic results for obesity treatment, credible information about its safety and effectiveness is simply not available.[58] The 1992 National Institutes of Health Technology Assessment Conference concluded that "Long term weight loss following any type of intervention was limited to only a small minority of the obese people studied."[59]

C. Wayne Callaway, an associate clinical professor of medicine at George Washington University, testifying at the 1990 congressional hearings for the American Board of Nutrition, said, "With rare exceptions, none of the popular commercially available programs for treating obesity is based on current scientific knowledge. (If they were), they could no longer promise rapid weight loss."[60]

When the National Institutes of Health and FDA requested data on the effectiveness of weight loss programs for the 1992 Technology Assessment Conference, they received research from only five companies. The studies of all but one were judged scientifically inadequate or inconclusive. The fifth company's 55 studies failed to show success in long-term weight loss.[61]

Some pediatric specialists, too, claim excellent results losing weight with children but, again, their data is weak. And research shows that most kids who are overweight — 60 percent of overweight 7-year-olds — will outgrow this stage without intervention, so this may be a factor in successes they do show.

The lack of properly trained professionals working with children in the weight loss industry is another concern. "Supervision of such programs varies from none, to instantly created certified counselors, to physicians with little or no training in this area, to a few physicians and registered dietitians and behavioral psychologists who truly have the required expertise," Callaway reported.

Why dieting doesn't work

The simple answer to why weight loss treatment doesn't work is that our bodies don't want it to. The human body defends its normal weight through a highly regulated internal system. Once this was called "setpoint" weight, but that term lost favor because some thought it meant predestined from birth.

I regard normal weight as the weight a person is now, at this time in life, when eating normally and not dieting. It results from a variety of genetic and environmental factors.

It's clear that this normal weight is being regulated. Just as the body monitors a consistent amount of salt in the blood (whether you eat more or less salt), and keeps body temperature steady (in a cold or warm room), so it adjusts to maintain normal weight. If you eat more calories than usual in a big holiday meal, your body works to get rid of the excess by increasing metabolism and body temperature and adjusting other factors, even appetite and satiety. If you eat less than usual, your body adjusts to conserve energy and promote increased eating.

That's why there are so many different methods to lose weight — because none of them really work. The faster a dieter loses weight, the faster weight is regained — two sides to the same coin.

Most nutritionists no longer believe in a simple numbers game, in which you can count calories in and calories out to figure pounds lost. It doesn't work over the long term — and if not, then why bother?

But yes, there are successes. I'm haunted by some of them — gaunt, hollow-eyed young women wholly focused on their day's meager allotment of food. Many stay thin through superhuman efforts that focus their lives around food, weight, and ways of denying hunger.

It makes you wonder, wouldn't they rather have a life?

For those eager to engage each new weight loss miracle, "just in case it works," my basic advice holds: Wait two years after the media and doctors and your friends are enthusiastically promoting this great miracle. In two years enthusiasm will have died down. You'll know the truth and will have saved yourself a lot of effort. So far it's proved good advice.

Certainly, for children and adolescents, it seems wise to delay. There's time to wait, and many years to regret a harmful decision.

The real successes that I'm seeing aim at improving lifestyle habits, changing gradually to living more actively, eating more moderately, relieving stress, and letting weight come off naturally (or not) as a result. Weight lost this way stays off because both habit and "set point" are changed.

But, unfortunately, most youngsters and adults want — and are continually being promised — the quick fix.

CHAPTER 9

New health approach needed

■

As these problems claim more and more children, it's time for a new approach. What we've been doing is not working well. Our children are afraid to eat. More are eating abnormally. More live with eating disorders. More struggle with overweight. More children and teens are contemplating suicide. More fail to thrive because of the social shame they endure for being fat.

While these problems are especially acute for American children, they are shared throughout the world.

It's time to throw out the old model. The traditional ways of dealing with weight and eating must be replaced by a new paradigm that helps children and does not harm them.

What we need to do is this: Consider the four eating and weight problems together as interrelated issues. We need to understand how they affect each other, and we need to be wary of the harm so easily done to vulnerable youth. Overweight, eating disorders, dysfunctional eating and size prejudice aren't separate issues, they're all part of the same problem and they're all influenced by our unnatural obsession with thinness.

In the new paradigm, we can deal with these issues in healthy ways.

The unified health approach

The goal of the new approach is the health and well-being of all children of all sizes, including their intellectual, physical, emotional, social and spiritual development.

To achieve this goal, a unified health approach is needed, as shown in the diagram on the facing page and the first chapter of this book. All children need to receive consistent messages which encourage normal eating, active living, self respect and an appreciation of size diversity. If they get these messages from national health policy, health care providers, teachers, their family and the media, then the four weight and eating problems can be prevented or diminished.

This new paradigm is about wellness and wholeness for every individual, and being healthy at the weight we are. It's about eating in normal, healthy ways, living actively, preventing problems, self acceptance, self respect and appreciation of diversity in others.

This is an approach that does no harm. Rather, the united effort acts on and responds to negative aspects of culture in positive and effective ways. It keeps a healthy perspective while challenging the detrimental effects of traditional thinking and health politics aimed at size alone.

We can help young people develop self respect, assertiveness and healthy coping skills. We can help them find their unique potential as lovable, capable, valuable individuals, so they will take pride in themselves and their bodies at whatever size they are.

This paradigm shifts the focus away from thinness to being healthy and active at our natural or normal weight. This is within everyone's reach.

There's much evidence that keeping a stable weight through adult life is healthy for persons of all sizes, much healthier than yo-yoing weight up and down, and that large people can be very healthy, of course. The risks of overweight have been greatly exaggerated (and the risks of underweight minimized).

Research suggests that fitness and activity may be more important than weight in determining good health and longevity. Steven Blair and his colleagues at the Cooper Institute for Aerobics Research in Dallas studied 25,389 men for more than eight years and

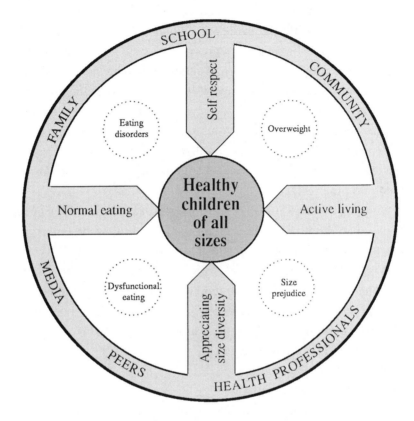

Figure 1

The unified health approach

To achieve the goal of healthy children of all sizes, a unified health approach is needed, whereby all children receive consistent messages which encourage normal eating, active living, self respect and an appreciation of size diversity. If family, teachers, health professionals, peers and the media give these messages to all children, the four major weight and eating problems (dysfunctional eating, eating disorders, overweight and size prejudice) will be diminished.

AFRAID TO EAT 1997

found disease and death rates were related to health behaviors, not fatness. At any weight, fit men outlived those with lower levels of fitness, and the fit obese men lived just as long as the fit lean men. Other studies suggest the same for women.[1]

The unified health approach grows out of the nondiet movement, led by people who advocate normal eating, active lifestyles, and stable weight, and reject the traditional thinking that everyone should be thin and that large people should always be trying to lose weight.

The new health paradigm unites the work of visionary people from many fields: nutrition, eating disorders, medicine, exercise science, obesity, psychology, size acceptance and others. It is research based and practical.

Many — perhaps most — nutritionists and dietitians now accept the new paradigm. They are among the first professionals to revise their traditional role in weight loss treatment. The new thinking is now reflected in policy decisions of the Society for Nutrition Education. That group has a special member section called Weight Realities that explores these issues. It is also reflected in American Dietetic Association position papers, and is widely accepted in Canadian nutrition and dietetics groups.

Changing national policy

By taking the unified health approach, we put all the issues on the table, recognizing that today's problems are not simple. They include obesity and its risks, the failure of weight loss treatment, pressures to be thin, the high rates of dysfunctional eating, malnutrition, dangerous weight loss methods, eating disorders, the stigmatizing of larger kids, and women's issues which impact body image for young girls. All these factors are in the mix when we consider the complex areas of weight and eating, and what they mean in our culture.

As shown earlier, healthy living is distorted when a single problem is the focus. Focusing on obesity intensifies other problems and self-esteem is damaged. An appalling example is the influential report *Weighing the Options,* which warns, "It is inappropriate to argue that obese individuals should simply accept their body weight and not try to reduce."[2]

Similarly, when the focus is solely on eating disorders, problems of excessive weight gain may be disregarded. When self respect is ignored, when we can't accept people who differ from the norm, when the power of society is brushed off, then we see more kids losing hope and contemplating suicide.

Emphasizing single issues sets one policy against another, and it violates the principle to do no harm.

Health professionals, educators and parents who are willing to look carefully at all the problems will find positive ways of working together to build strengths in all these areas.

Taking a broader view and recognizing reality is especially important for those who set national health policy. They need to drop the fiction that weight loss treatment programs are working. They must add eating disorders to the health agenda in Healthy People 2010. Only then, when all the issues are allowed on the table, can a comprehensive policy be developed which makes sense and which health professionals will support.

Changing national policy in the U.S., which I fully expect to follow the recognition of eating disorders, will bring about a major improvement, since it sets the agenda for what happens throughout

---

The unified health paradigm

The unified health approach helps prevent weight and eating problems through encouraging:

- Self trust and empowerment
- Normal eating balanced by active living
- Normal growth for children, stable weight for adults
- Self acceptance and self respect
- An appreciation of size diversity, tolerance, and respect for others

The new paradigm embraces the Canadian *Vitality* message:

Enjoy eating well, being active and feeling good about yourself.

AFRAID TO EAT 1997

the country. National policy also greatly influences how the media reports health issues.

This happened in Canada, where a shift in policy has brought a remarkable shift in schools, community and health care.

The opposing debate

Arguments against this new health paradigm are lodged in the concern that if the public is allowed to lose its fear of fat and accept size diversity, we'll see a tremendous increase in overweight. Further, that even though current obesity treatments don't work and can cause harm, the public needs to keep believing in them, because someday there will be drugs that work and people must be kept in a mood to take them. And there's fear the weight loss industry may be damaged by a more open approach.

These are weak arguments based on fallacies, not research or reality, in my opinion. First, the fear of fat has not prevented obesity; it has likely exacerbated it during the last 15 or 20 years by causing increased dysfunctional eating. Second, the public will recognize and respond to honesty in an area where it has so often been deceived. It is untrue that the new paradigm opposes obesity treatment. Rather, when safe and effective treatment is available, it will fit well into this sound, healthy approach and size-accepting people will certainly use it when appropriate. Third, yes, there may indeed be loss of profits for weight loss companies, but those willing to develop worthwhile lifestyle programs can benefit.

How to enact changes

So how can we do this? How can we develop a shared vision and consistent messages that communicate this vision?

Healthy lifestyle programs fit well into the new approach by shifting emphasis away from weight loss and toward self trust, empowerment, self acceptance, and the prevention of problems. This new approach encourages children to eat, move and grow in normal ways, working with their natural regulatory abilities. It promotes natural, wholesome eating patterns, healthy food relationships and regular physical activities. It sets the stage in childhood for healthy lifestyles that will enable individuals to maintain a natural, stable weight through life.

Ellyn Satter, MS, RD, a registered dietitian, family therapist and well-known authority on feeding infants and children, explains that the emerging paradigm is based on trusting our bodies and accepts that fatness may be normal for some people, unlike the current "control paradigm" that assumes all obesity is harmful and must be fixed. "The task for the growing child is not to remain slim, but to maintain energy balance in response to variations in caloric density of the diet, activity level and growth."

"It means listening to your body," writes Linda Omichinski, author of *You Count, Calories Don't* and *Teens and Diets: No Weigh.* "It means discovering individual patterns for food and activity levels that keep you energized. It means finding the strength to accept yourself just as you are and get on with life."

Programs based on the new paradigm offer a fresh approach that is flexible, open, accepting, individualized and family-centered.

Leaders in the new programs recognize that parents are confused and shaken by today's conflicting health messages and need to trust in themselves again. New programs appreciate local culture and values. Parents are assured they can trust their family traditions, that traditional foods and ways of celebrating with food are valuable to pass down through the generations, shaped and expressed in different ways as they may be, yet honoring the past. They learn to trust their own judgment and feel confident that they and their children can make good decisions.

The message is "trust yourself." Trust and empower the child. Support the child in solving his or her own problems, even when that child marches to a different drummer.

A new definition

Satter suggests the new definition of obesity should be fatness that is abnormal or unnecessary for the individual. Fatness may be just as normal for children at the heaviest 5 percent as thinness is for the lightest 5 percent, if they show a consistent and predictable pattern of growth, and any growth adjustments are gradual and occur over time. If fatness is the result of unstable body weight with abrupt or acute weight gain, it is likely to be abnormal, she says.

Satter believes that children who are grounded in their internal regulatory processes are more likely to avoid eating errors and to sustain appropriate body weight regulation throughout life.

A leader in the new paradigm, Satter has untiringly presented her innovative ideas to nutrition leaders for more than a decade, inspiring many to move in new directions. In 1987 she published her ground-breaking book, *How to Get Your Kid to Eat . . . But Not Too Much,* expanding on ideas presented in her 1983 book, *Child of Mine.*[3]

Does the new paradigm work?

Whether or not it "works" depends on the outcome goal, Satter explains. "If the goal is to help children grow in a stable and consistent fashion and achieve the adult body that is right for them, then, yes, the emerging paradigm works. What results from such humanistic and realistic strategies is normal growth. And normal growth works.

"If the goal of preventive intervention with children's weight is the current one of keeping children from growing up fat, probably not. But the current paradigm proponents haven't kept children thin, either, even when they try harder. In fact, trying to externally control food intake and activity can undermine children's ability to maintain energy balance and make them fatter than they otherwise would be.

"Children have their own considerable capability with eating, activity and growth and the best approach is to support that capability rather than trying to outwit it. Working with rather than against these natural regulatory abilities enhances the likelihood of maintaining stable body weight throughout life."

The new programs understand and deal with the current youth crisis, in which many girls have arrested their intellectual and physical development in trying desperately to reshape their bodies.

Moving ahead

This new way of dealing with weight and eating issues is moving ahead. We are in the midst of a new movement that will not be stopped. The response is everywhere positive to this new approach.

Diets that don't work, pressures to be thin, and the crisis in disturbed eating — are all reasons why women and men are responding with enthusiasm.

Women are in the forefront of this new movement. And this is as it should be. Women know the issues. They are well aware how disproportionately young girls suffer from eating disorders, dysfunctional eating, and the stigma of overweight. They have struggled with their own weight and body issues. And they are concerned that boys and men not suffer as women have suffered.

There is even a feminist perspective to all this, although most of these committed women do not call themselves feminists. They hold that dieting and semi-starvation keep women preoccupied and passive, away from career ambitions, and that women are dehumanized by their portrayal in the media, advertising and the fashion industry.

These visionary women, naturally, are joined by supportive and visionary men. Mostly they are professionals in health and wellness fields. They are educators, extension agents, writers, researchers, health providers, mothers and fathers. These leaders are committed to changing our culture, to speaking out, challenging, sometimes boycotting what exceeds the bounds of being nurturing toward children in our society.

Growing up large is acceptable

Leaders in the new movement are committed to helping people understand that the body cannot be shaped at will. That individual differences in body shapes and sizes are natural and desirable. That the weight which evolves naturally from healthy lifestyle needs to be accepted.

And yes, the new leaders are willing to accept what has long been unacceptable: that obese youngsters may not achieve permanent weight loss or grow up to be thin. The new guidelines and programs recognize this and deal with it in a straightforward manner.

"There is no reason your child cannot lead a happy, productive, full life at whatever size she turns out to be," explains Joanne Ikeda, MA, RD, a California nutrition education specialist with the Cooperative Extension Service, University of California, Berkeley, and

The shift to *Vitality* from a
weight centered approach

Weight centered approach	VITALITY
DIETING	**HEALTHY EATING**
• Restrictive eating • Counting calories, prescriptive diets • Weight cycling (yo-yo diets) • Eating disorders	• Take pleasure in eating a variety of foods • Enjoy lower-fat, complex-carbohydrate foods more often • Meet the body's energy and nutrient needs through a lifetime of healthy, enjoyable eating • Take control of how you eat by listening to your hunger cues
EXERCISE	**ACTIVE LIVING**
• No pain, no gain • Prescriptions such as three times a week in your target heart-rate zone • Burn calories • High attrition rates for exercise programs	• Value and practice activities that are moderate and fun • Be active your way, every day • Participate for the joy of feeling your body move • Enjoy physical activities as part of your daily lifestyle
DISSATISFACTION WITH SELF	**POSITIVE SELF/BODY IMAGE**
• Unrealistic goals for body size and shape • Obsession and preoccupation with weight • Fat phobia and discrimination against overweight people • Striving to be a perfect "10" and to maintain an impossible "ideal" (thin or muscular) body size • Accepting the fashion, diet and tobacco industries' emphasis on slimness	• Accept and recognize that healthy bodies come in a range of weights, shapes/sizes • Appreciate your strengths and abilities • Be tolerant of a wide range of body sizes and shapes • Relax and enjoy the unique characteristics you have to offer • Be critical of messages that focus on unrealistic thinness (in women) and muscularity (in men) as symbols of success and happiness

The VITALITY approach calls for a shift from negative to positive thinking about how to achieve and maintain healthy weight.[2]

VITALITY/HEALTHY WEIGHT JOURNAL MAY/JUN 1995/AFRAID TO EAT 1997 leader in the size acceptance movement.

In the brochure *If My Child is Overweight, What should I do about it?,* Ikeda tells parents, "Being overweight may seem like the worst possible fate. However, it isn't. A worse fate is feeling rejected and unloved because one is overweight.[4]

"You can make sure this does not happen to your child. Reassure your child she will be loved by you always, whether she is thin or fat. Help your child to feel good about herself so that overweight is not compounded by low self-esteem."

Canada's *Vitality* program puts it this way: "To overcome the influence of a media-dominated culture that judges women on how they look, we must encourage women to accept a wide range of healthy body weights and shapes, to love their bodies as they are, to value slimness only as it relates to overall health, to refrain from dieting and to reject societal pressures to conform to an unrealistic body size. In doing so, women will improve their self-images and be more realistic in their assessment of body image.

"One of the results of living in a thinness culture is the belief that health is improved with weight loss and achieving a low body weight. This basic assumption has been challenged and the negative effects of dieting and weight cycling are now being examined closely.

"While a reduction in weight will improve the health of some overweight people, a fixation on weight reduction and ideal body shape can lead to yo-yo dieting, weight cycling, restrictive eating, obsessive exercising and negative perceptions of body image. Furthermore, pursuit of a rigid standard for size and shape inevitably fails for most people over the long term."[5]

Networking and learning together

It's been my privilege to network with many of these new leaders through 12 years of writing, editing and publishing *Healthy Weight Journal.* I've been inspired by their new, healthier approaches to problems, and gratified when they are inspired by my ideas and insights.

We have a lot to learn, and I've learned, from scientists and specialists in obesity, eating disorders and related fields. My memberships in an eclectic clutch of professional organizations — in the fields of obesity, eating disorders, nutrition, health, size acceptance and health fraud — have helped me understand the differing viewpoints. I attend their conferences, listen, present, review their diverse literature and research, study their journals and newsletters, talk by telephone, e-mail and face-to-face with specialists, researchers, teachers, and ordinary people with problems. All have poignant and powerful information to share.

Canadian educators and health professionals have achieved what we in the U.S. have not yet been able to do: they've changed national policy. Health Canada now encourages a national way of thinking that focuses on health instead of weight. I began talking with leaders in the Canadian movement in the mid-1980s. They discovered me first as readers of *Healthy Weight Journal*, and started sending their innovative ideas my way. It's been an awakening experience.

Heather Nielsen, Chief of Nutrition Programs at Health Canada in Ottawa, first sent me papers from a series of health policy meetings that discussed obesity along with eating disorders, preoccupation with weight and negative body image. It was a new way to advance knowledge I hadn't seen before. As an important part of the decision-making team, they included female eating disorder specialists who embrace the new paradigm. In the U.S., such specialists are seldom included in health policy planning.

Then these bold Canadians tore apart the sacrosanct height-weight charts we've always used and worked out broader ranges. Finally, they more or less shelved the "healthy weight" ranges, too, and after months and years of meetings by eminent specialists in various fields, they settled on a single eloquent concept: *Vitality*. Vitality is simplicity itself. It tells Canadians and people all over the world: "Enjoy eating well, being active and feeling good about yourself."

Vitality is an integrated approach to healthy living that shifts the focus away from rigid goals, dieting and prescriptive exercise toward the acceptance of a range of body sizes and shapes and an emphasis on healthy eating, active living and positive self and body image. Vitality encourages us to be healthy at the weight we are, get on with life, and stop obsessing about weight. It's a message of preventing problems before they happen. It is also the basis for new treatment programs with its three-pronged approach of eating well, living actively and self-esteem. School programs emphasize nondieting, eating normally, improving self-esteem and dealing with size discrimination.

I've been so enthusiastic about Vitality, that at one point Heather Nielsen and I went to Washington, D.C, where I was pleased and honored be able to set up a presentation for a nutrition group and invited public health officials. The nutritionists loved the challenging new ideas, but it had no discernible effect on health policy. Maybe we planted seeds. But it seemed to me, rather, that the new ideas may have posed a threat to power and strengthened resistance to change within a closed circle.

My awareness has been greatly expanded, too, by leaders in the size acceptance movement, who years ago began sending me information and including me in their communications. Getting to know size activist leaders from the U.S., England, Australia and other countries has been enlightening. It's also been a delight and surprise to have become a rallying point for size acceptance groups from around the world after we began a regular feature that showcases their viewpoint in *Healthy Weight Journal*. Their increasingly articulate views have been important in shaping national debate.

A better vision

Working together and supported by a unified health policy that deals with weight and eating issues, we can bring about the healthy change needed for our children and our future.

As we search for answers, it is important to keep a balanced perspective. We need to remember that weight, eating and health are only part of what makes life worthwhile. Wellness and wholeness are not about attaining perfect health or even longevity, but improving our quality of life, so we live well emotionally, intellectually, physically, socially and spiritually.

In the family, caring parents or significant others who understand the issues set the stage with unconditional love and acceptance, no matter what, from infancy on. They give reassurance that every child is okay, just as he or she is, and they model and teach normal eating, active living and a positive outlook on life.

Schools provide the intellectually stimulating environment needed for learning when they are safe and accepting — safe from emotional violence, harassment and bullying, and safe from physical violence. And students, in turn, gain most from the academic process when they are well nourished, with minds ready to learn, not focused on food, hunger, weight or appearance.

Ways to integrate school and community health programs are being rediscovered. For example, communities across the country are finding new energy by working through a Minneapolis-based program called "Healthy Communities, Healthy Youth" by the Search Institute. Goals are to create an environment in which all young people are valued, problems become manageable, and an attitude of vision, hope and celebration pervades community life.[6]

Programs like this motivate communities to ensure a child-friendly culture through existing organizations and institutions. They emphasize a unified positive approach, so that instead of looking at problems in a negative way, communities shift toward effective preventive action.

As we embrace this new approach, we need to make changes in five major areas: attitude, lifestyle, prevention, health care and knowledge. Shifting toward a unified health approach in these areas will further the goal of raising healthy children of all sizes. It will free our children, and help them live happy, productive, fulfilling lives.

CHAPTER 10

In the family

■

Families are a critical, positive force in defusing this public health crisis. Parents or other significant adults in their lives can help children restore normal eating, and the sooner, the better. The longer they struggle with eating and weight issues, the more dysfunctional these can become. And the more likely that the issues will deteriorate into more severe problems. If an eating disorder is suspected it's important to have the problem evaluated by a competent therapist and if needed, get the child into therapy without delay.

Yet it is easy to add to the anxiety, fear and pressure these kids are already feeling. A flexible, low-key approach focusing on supporting the child with love and acceptance helps reduce tensions.

Families today take many different structures. Blended or single-parent families are as common as the traditional two parent household. What's important is that families with healthy attitudes and behavior are at the heart of promoting healthy growth and development for their children.

Mothers, fathers or significant others in children's lives who are obsessed or worried over their own weight, continually dieting, restricting fat or calories, and often talking about these concerns, can set children up for eating problems at very young ages. A parent's overconcern about a child's weight further adds to the tension, fear and confusion a child is feeling.

It's important for families to be safe places where children are loved and accepted unconditionally, as beautiful and capable individuals. But often parents don't know how to deal with a child who is struggling with dysfunctional eating, an eating disorder, overweight or size prejudice.

Children are crying out for help and support from their families. I receive heartbreaking letters from teenagers who are struggling to cope with weight and eating pressures in their lives. Many of them write about communicating: I can't talk to my parents; they're too busy; they won't listen; they don't understand; they want to run my life; they say it's nothing, to forget it.

What can I tell them? I'm a parent and I've made mistakes. I'm not a therapist.

But I tell them you are lovable, beautiful and capable just as you are. I hope you'll come to accept yourself, and believe in yourself. Learning acceptance will help release the tension that you say is taking over your life and threatening to tear apart your family. And please stop those thoughts of suicide. You said you didn't want to hurt your parents, but this is a way to hurt them badly for the rest of their lives. You can interrupt your negative thoughts and replace them with pleasant images if you'll work on it. I hope you will.

Find someone to talk to — your parents, a therapist, school counsellor, pastor or priest, friend. Talking about how you feel will help.

It's sad that you, and kids like you, are being made to feel you have to meet some ridiculous standard to be loved and accepted. I hope our nation will soon rediscover its appreciation of diversity and stop focusing on physical appearance.

You're okay just as you are. Tall is nice, short is nice — so is large or small, or being attractive or not so attractive. This is the way life is. It's us, all of us, the human race in all its wonderful diversity.

I know this tolerance is not being shown right now, especially in the media, and I'm sorry about that. But I have faith it will change. You and I, your mom and dad, our friends, working together, we can bring about changes to make our culture safe, secure and accepting for all.

Family communication

It's important that families talk to each other, especially about feelings. Some parents don't know how to express their feelings or are afraid. They're afraid they'll be unable to help or know the right answers, so they discourage their children from talking about their own feelings.

Communication builds relationships. It lets moms and dads know what their kids are doing and thinking. It helps kids understand who their parents are. It lays a foundation for positive family life. And it helps kids deal with scary things going on in their lives — transitions to the next grade or from elementary school to junior high school, divorce, separation, discouragement or grief.

It's helpful if moms and dads will ask, "How do you feel about that?" and then listen, without offering advice. In fact, trying to solve problems that should be "owned" by the child can be controlling and destructive behavior for parents. Instead, helpful parents will listen in a caring way, and trust the child to explore solutions.

The foundation for free and open expression is laid in childhood. As they get older, kids still want to talk to parents about their problems and freely express their feelings, but don't want them taken over and "solved," or belittled. This is especially important for teenagers, who soon stop sharing when this happens.

Sometimes a problem seems small to the parent — a torn favorite shirt, a friend's snub, missing out on an event. Enabling them to talk it out can help children keep it small and let it go. It can help them diffuse anxiety or anger and deal with it in constructive ways. Or it may uncover other, larger problems that need attention.

Sometimes the problem looms so large for the entire family that it is believed too terrible to talk about: alcoholism, financial losses, marital discord, an unfortunate experience, or physical, sexual or mental abuse.

Children need to know it's okay to talk about these things, even when hurtful. That it's not a good situation, but mom has feelings she can talk about, so does dad, and so does each of the children. When nothing is ever said, the terrible problem grows even worse.

In the case of sexual molestation, it will help children if they know they don't have to put up with this. Too often this is not clear to them. Giving them the words to use and practicing it loud and clear can help: "Don't do that, I don't like it." (This is not to suggest this is the child's problem, it isn't. Parents and the community are responsible for protecting children from physical, mental and sexual abuse. But it happens, and being prepared can help.)

Pretending everything is perfect in the home and conveying the idea that, above all, the family must look perfect in the eyes of neighbors, sets an impossible standard. It causes enormous stress and sets children up for many kinds of emotional problems.

This stress may be expressed in eating disturbances and disorders. Talking about it and expressing feelings diffuses the stress and helps children cope in healthier ways.

Parents who are "too busy" to listen and disengaged parents who don't try may want to do some soul-searching about what is really important in their lives. Finding the time and energy to listen at the time it is most needed may be difficult, but it is extremely important in children's lives. On the other hand, some parents are too controlling, too involved. If they will back off, they can empower their children by trusting them to make their own decisions.

It's all part of parenting, giving our children roots and wings.

Caring neighbors

One of the greatest resources for young people is having ongoing relationships with caring, principled people outside the home. Adults who offer guidance and encouragement, who care about and trust them. They gain much strength from support across the generations, by hearing consistent messages about boundaries and values from neighbors, relatives, older and younger adults from school, church and community, adults who call them by name and are their friends.

Many children and teens are missing this support network today. In a Minneapolis study, only 29 percent of youth reported having caring neighbors. Many adults have pulled back from offering their support to neighborhood kids because they feel overwhelmed by frightening youth problems that dominate the headlines. Often neighbors don't get involved in the lives of children on their block, and may not even know their names. Instead of offering support, they defer problems to professionals.

The Search Institute in Minneapolis turns this around by urging people to take action on their own. Through the "Healthy Communities, Healthy Youth" program, adults are encouraged to do simple things: look at and speak to every child or teen you see; talk to youngsters about their interests; send a birthday or congratulatory card; invite a young person to go along to a ballgame; have an open-door policy so neighbor kids feel welcome to come in for conversation, refreshments, or just hang out.[1]

Everyone gets involved. In some Search communities, senior citizens wait for school buses with children, making sure they're safely off to school, while building relationships with children they didn't know before. Girls on the basketball team read to younger children in the library on Saturdays. All residents see themselves as guardians of the community's young people. It's a positive action to reverse the crumbling infrastructure of neighborhoods all across the country.

Towns, communities, and the entire state of Colorado are taking advantage of this program to break through barriers. The rewards of rebuilding the sense of neighborhood and caring will last for generations.

Building assets for children

Search focuses on 40 assets, or building blocks, to help promote the healthy development of children. Surveys show that the more of these assets young people have, the more they engage in positive behaviors, such as volunteering and succeeding in school. The fewer they have, the more likely they engage in risk-taking behaviors, such as violence, sexual activity, alcohol and drug use. Each asset is important, and together the benefits are additive.

The goal of a Search community is to increase the number of each child's assets. Examples of these assets include:

- Support from three or more non-parent adults.
- Caring neighbors.
- Active, involved parents.
- An attachment to school.

- Desire to help other people.
- Commitment to serve in your community.
- Training in music and the arts.
- Religious participation.
- Skills to resolve conflict nonviolently.
- Optimism about your personal future.

Children, their families and their neighbors all know these 40 assets and strive to increase them for every young person.

This is the kind of action that can bring about healthier families, schools and communities and a child-nurturing, supportive culture for our youth.

Being aware of the benefits of this kind of network of caring adults who nurture their children can help parents feel supported. Building and nourishing these relationships is a vital task of parenting. It's especially important now when kids are so heavily influenced by pop culture and the entertainment industries.

The community approach provides families with a supportive, caring network of friends in raising their children. It creates the kind of informal associations that previous generations of parents depended on for support and guidance.

The asset-building Search approach helps parents. Parents feel supported. The local media repeatedly communicate the vision in these communities, support local mobilization efforts, and provide forums for sharing innovative actions.

"The community is filled with consistent messages," says Peter Benson, president of Search Institute. "If you spend time in an asset-building community, you quickly sense harmony in the messages that young people hear . . . People consistently hear that young people are a priority in the community."

Restore normal lifestyles

An emphasis on sound, healthy lifestyles is the best known prevention for weight and eating problems of all kinds. As in the Canadian Vitality healthy weight programs, a healthy family focus will be on eating well, living actively and feeling good about yourself.

"Vitality is a shift in thinking about what healthy living really is.

It's a lifestyle for everyone. It's throwing a Frisbee with the kids, having friends over for a potluck dinner, curling up enjoying a good book. It's about healthy eating and active living. It's gardening and cycling, laughing and relaxing. It's good for you — body and soul."

Mothers, fathers and children who feel good about themselves and each other make healthy choices easy — not just for a short period of time but for a lifetime.

Restoring normal eating is a priority for those who have restricted their eating and for those who habitually overeat. Unfortunately, to-day many parents are so confused and fearful of their own eating, weight and health, that their fears are multiplied in their children. They need to realize that their own attitudes and behaviors may contribute to their children's eating and weight problems.

Normal eating

Normal eating is distinguished by regular eating habits. It is regu-lated for the most part by internal signals of hunger, appetite and satiety. Normal eating enhances our feelings of well-being. Normal eating nurtures good health, vibrant energy, and the healthy growth and development of children. Food choices provide variety, modera-tion, and balanced nutrition. Normal eating promotes clear thinking, the ability to concentrate, mood stability and healthy relationships with family, friends and community.

People who eat normally will not all be thin. They exhibit a range of stable weights, as their normal weight is expressed through a variety of inherited and environmental factors.

Normal eating is described in terms of self-trust, flexibility and responding to body signals by Ellyn Satter in *How to Get Your Kid to Eat . . . But Not Too Much.*[2]

"Normal eating is being able to eat when you are hungry and continue eating until you are satisfied. It is being able to choose food you like and eat it and truly get enough of it — not just stop eating because you think you should. Normal eating is being able to use some moderate constraint in your food selection to get the right food, but not being so restrictive that you miss out on pleasurable foods.

"Normal eating is giving yourself permission to eat sometimes

Developing positive eating habits

Which will you do?

Instead of . . .	Try this
Using food as a reward or bribe	Give hugs and kisses instead of food
Letting your child drink from a bottle	Have your child use a cup
Letting your child eat whenever he wants	Set regular meal and snack times
Letting your child eat whatever he wants	Offer a choice of healthful foods
Quieting your child with food	Comfort your child with attention and affection
Setting stricter limits for larger child than rest of the family	Use the same limits and foods for all members of family
Letting your child help himself/herself to food	Store food out of sight and out of reach
Letting your child watch TV or play with toys during mealtime	Take away distractions during mealtime

Developed by the Wisconsin Department of Health and Social Services. Adapted from Child of Mine, *by Ellyn Satter, and* Your Growing Child, *by the California Department of Health Services.*[1]

because you are happy, sad or bored, or just because it feels good. Normal eating is three meals a day, most of the time, but it can also be choosing to munch along . . . Normal eating is trusting your body to make up for your mistakes in eating.

"In short, normal eating is flexible. It varies in response to your emotions, your schedule, your hunger, and your proximity to food."

Normal eating is not about rules, but developing reasonable habits that allow us to put eating in a comfortable groove and get on with life. It will differ for different individuals — we each need to find what works, trusting ourselves, and make it a habit. Habits are useful because, like brushing your teeth or fastening your seatbelt, once it has become a habit you don't waste time or mental energy thinking about it; you just do it.

Normal eating differs from abnormal or dysfunctional eating in that the latter is irregular and chaotic, out of synch with body needs, often aimed at reshaping the body. Thoughts and decisions about food, hunger, and weight can occupy 20 to 65 percent of waking hours. Instead of feeling better after eating, the person may feel worse — ashamed, guilty, anxious or uncomfortably full. It is common to feel fatigued, irritable, moody, chilled, unable to concentrate.

Positive feeding

Satter says it is essential for parents to maintain a positive feeding relationship through the growing up years that will allow kids to feel relaxed and comfortable about eating and in touch with their internal cues of hunger, appetite and satiety. Underfeeding interferes with this, just as surely as does urging a child to eat more than he or she wants.

She teaches a *Golden Rule for Parenting with Food:*

"Parents are responsible for what is presented to eat and the manner in which it is presented. Children are responsible for how much and even whether they eat."

This means that parents should select and buy food for the family, put meals on the table, have meals and snacks at regular times, and serve the food in a positive and supportive fashion. Then they need to trust the child to decide which foods and how much of each

Normal eating

What is normal eating?

■ Normal eating is distinguished by regular eating habits, typically three meals a day and snacks to satisfy hunger. It is regulated mostly by internal signals of hunger, appetite, satiety — we eat when hungry and stop when satisfied.

How does it promote health and well-being?

■ Normal eating enhances our feelings of well-being. We eat for health and energy, also for pleasure and social reasons, and afterward, we feel good.

■ Normal eating means that food choices more likely provide variety, moderation, and balanced nutrition.

■ Normal eating promotes clear thinking and mood stability. It fosters healthy relationships in family, work, school, and community. Thoughts of food, hunger, weight occupy only a small part of day (perhaps 10 to 15 percent).

■ Normal eating nurtures good health, vibrant energy, and the healthy growth and development of children. It promotes stable weights, within a wide range, expressing both genetic and environmental factors.

How does it differ from dysfunctional eating?

■ Dysfunctional or disordered eating patterns are irregular and chaotic (fasting, bingeing, dieting, skipping meals), or may mean usually overeating or undereating much more or less than the body wants or needs. Instead of feeling better after eating, the person is likely to feel worse.

■ Feeling fatigued, irritable, moody, chilled, less able to concentrate, and increasingly self-absorbed is common. Thoughts of food, hunger, and weight may occupy 20 to 65 percent of waking hours, or more. Potential health problems vary depending on the dysfunction. Risk of developing eating disorders is increased.

How parents encourage normal eating

1. Offer a variety of nutritious food at regular intervals — planned meals and snacks.
2. Help the child identify hunger and fullness.
3. Be a good example of normal, healthy eating and lifestyle.
4. Follow Ellyn Satter's *Golden Rule for Parenting with Food:*
   a. Parents are responsible for what is presented to eat and the manner in which it is presented.
   b. Children are responsible for how much and even whether they eat.

AFRAID TO EAT 1997

he or she will eat. This is the child's responsibility, Satter explains, and parents should not interfere with the eating process by urging, bribing, scolding or praising for eating. Let children eat like children and eat as much as they want. Allowing children to freely make their own decisions about food lets them respond appropriately to their internal cues of hunger and satiety.

Unfortunately, this natural division of responsibility is often violated by parents with rigid or restricting eating styles of their own, who try to take over their children's eating, who urge them to eat more, to clean their plates — or to stop eating before they are satisfied. This sets the stage for disruptive and disturbed eating patterns.

Satter says it is sometimes hard to convince parents that "Even the fat child is entitled to regulate the amount of food he eats."

Mothers and fathers have three responsibilities in feeding children, according to Iowa State University specialists, Carol Hans, RD, Extension Nutritionist, and Diane Nelson, Extension Communication Specialist.[3]

- ■ Offering the child a variety of nutritious foods at regular intervals. Planned meals and snacks give the child regular sources of energy, help the child develop sensible eating patterns, and encourage positive food behavior in social situations.

- ■ Helping the child identify and pay attention to feelings of hunger and fullness. This starts with learning to distinguish a baby's hungry cry from other cries. It means not urging a toddler to eat one more bite. It means sometimes having second or third helpings.

- ■ Demonstrating a healthy lifestyle. Children learn by example and are likely to do what parents do, whether it is eating chips while watching television, or going bicycling after supper.

Family meals eaten at home help to structure children's eating in healthy ways. In eating together, families gain a better sense of themselves and moral values are shared in a pleasant, relaxed setting. All this, yes, with the television turned off so families can relate to each other and catch up on events without distraction.

Eating together has many benefits.

"Family meals establish traditions and create pleasant memories as members discuss events of the day. Teens benefit greatly from this time together," says Kathy Walsh, Wells County extension agent in Harvey, N.D., and mother of three. "Meals promote communication skills, cooperation, cooking skills and table manners. (And) children who eat meals with their parents and siblings tend to eat a more varied and nutritious diet. Let the kids help prepare the meal and they are more likely to eat it. If this is a new idea to your family, give it a try . . . it could surprise you and provide some great memories."[4]

For families on the run, Walsh suggests being creative and flexible. "Bring the family together for a late dessert or eat breakfast together. Make weekend meals the family focus."

The dieting child

How can parents help when a teenager is determined to lose weight?

Sometimes all moms and dads can do is go along, help as they can, and ease the stress. Decisions on what and how much to eat belong to the child; this cannot be infringed.

As a parent of wrestlers, I understand this all too well. High school wrestling is a great sport and I enjoy it. But losing too much weight is a major problem that needs fixing in many schools. Our two sons were champion wrestlers in the lower weights and they believed that to be champions they had to lose a lot of weight.

With our oldest son Rick, I did everything wrong. His single-minded purpose was so devastating, his level of nutrition so low, and his eating so chaotic, that I felt helpless. I was a nutrition teacher, but I didn't know what to do.

Rick ate candy bars nonstop and hot dogs at the gym after a match. The next day he'd eat big meals with lots of cookies and snacks, then back to almost nothing, even restricting water the day or two before the next match. The rest of our family ate as usual. We'd try to coax him to meals, but mostly we tiptoed around and tried not to notice. He'd be kind of irritable after a hard workout, and we learned to leave him alone in that mood.

Now I understand that being irritable and moody is a classic, textbook reaction to hunger and malnutrition.

One day when he came home from school I had just baked brownies. I took them out of the oven about the time Rick came in and the house was full of good baking smells.

He walked into the kitchen — and I'll never forget the expression of rage, frustration and despair in his face. "You baked brownies! How can you do this to me?"

That really hurt. I was trying to be a good mother and keep goodies in the house for the rest of the family. But he was right. Instead of helping him, I was tempting him with just the kind of non-nutritive food he didn't need.

With our younger son Mike it was easier. I fixed the same small nutrient-dense meals for all of us, no frills, with limited fat and sugars. He still ate almost nothing those two days before matches, but otherwise ate quite well.

One of the tough things about high school wrestling season is that it comes during both Thanksgiving and Christmas holidays. A mother whose three sons were wrestling told me that they hadn't had a Christmas dinner in 10 years that one of the boys didn't rush from the table in tears, run upstairs and slam his bedroom door.

We normally celebrate with traditional holiday dinners, and a bountiful table. But when Mike was wrestling I'd fill plates in the kitchen, spreading out the food so it looked like more, offer fewer choices to reduce temptations, and add big no-calorie gelatin salads. They weren't great meals and I knew Mike's thoughts were on the turkey in the kitchen, but we tried to make them fun.

Yet the night Mike won the state championship at 105 pounds, he probably should have had another 10 or 20 pounds just for endurance — and his opponent was in much the same shape. It still hurts to see that gaunt-faced photo of Mike with his trophy.

Reassurance on size

It's natural for parents to want their children to be as perfect as possible, but when it comes to weight, "perfect" must be broadly and individually defined, advise Hans and Nelson. In their brochure, *A Parent's Guide to Children's Weight,* they remind parents that children grow at different rates and may have very different body structures from their own brothers and sisters.

"Ideally, parents help their children learn to recognize their own feelings of hunger and choose appropriate, nutritious foods to satisfy hunger. They also can help the child learn to see food as only one of many possible ways to celebrate a happy event, to ease disappointment, or to erase boredom."

Hans and Nelson advise parents that a child who is too thin needs the same emotional support as one who is too heavy. A visit to a pediatrician can help put the child's size in perspective and provide a basis for reminding children that individuals grow at different rates. And parents can refrain from comment about their children's size or shape, except in a reassuring way.

When a child shows a sudden weight drop, other medical or emotional problems may be suspected. Professional help from a pediatrician, dietitian or child psychologist may be necessary.

Beyond reassuring the large child of parental love regardless of his or her weight, the appropriate parental action depends on whether the whole family has lifestyle problems. If the family needs to change some eating and exercise habits, then parent and child can work together to initiate and plan those changes for everyone's benefit.

"For example, many social traditions are related to food and eating, such as giving food as a reward for completing a task, as a sympathetic gesture to ease hurt feelings, or as a cure for boredom," say Hans and Nelson. "These habits may lead the child to expect food in those situations, regardless of any feelings of hunger. By helping the child learn that such behavior is occasional, the child may avoid forming some of the dependent habits that can cause later weight problems."

If the child is the only family member with a weight problem, possible medical problems or emotional stresses need to be considered.

"Since a parent's primary role is to give support, any action that denies support should be avoided," say Hans and Nelson. "For example, when a child is upset by playmates' teasing, a parent who responds with, 'When you get thinner they won't tease you any-more,' only reinforces the child's suspicion that there is indeed some-thing wrong with him or her. A more positive response is for the parent to listen to the child express his or her feelings about that teasing, and then perhaps, ask if other children are getting teased and for what reason. This can lead to a discussion of: 'What do you think you can do about this situation?'"

Parents should not treat the overweight child differently, such as giving one child different meals, desserts or snacks from the rest of the family, they point out. Similarly, putting the child on a weight loss diet is a form of punishment that asks them to ignore feelings of hunger and may lead them to believe there is truly something wrong for wanting to eat more than their parents want to give them.

Family coping with eating disorders

Parents who are concerned that a child may have an eating dis-order or severe eating problems should see their family doctor, dieti-tian or an eating disorder specialist.

An adolescent may feel very uncomfortable talking about his or her eating, and refuse to see a professional. Try negotiating, suggests Stephanie Fortin, MA, a Canadian eating disorder specialist in the *National Eating Disorder Information Centre Bulletin.*[5] Negotiate slowly, one step at a time, while reassuring her of your concern for her health and well-being, rather than demanding she enter treatment.

The National Eating Disorders Organization suggests the careful selection of a therapist, and advises patients, "You have the right to choose the gender of your therapist; you have the right to ask to talk with the therapist ahead of time to clarify his or her experience in this area and treatment approach. Listen to your feelings . . . If you feel you can work well with this person, then make a commitment to treatment."

NEDO offers reassurance that recovery can take time. "Working through an eating disorder is very difficult, an 'up and down' pro-cess." Relapse back to baseline or worse is a recognized pattern in eating disorder treatment, even after seemingly successful treatment.

Preventing eating disorders

Ten things parents can do

by Linda Smolak and Michael P. Levine

1. Avoid conveying an attitude about yourself or your children which proclaims "I will like you more if you lose weight, eat less, wear a smaller size, eat only 'good' foods." Avoid negative statements about your own body and your own eating.

2. Educate yourself and your children about (a) the genetic basis of differences in body shapes and body weight; and (b) the nature and ugliness of prejudice. Be certain that your child understands that weight gain is a normal and necessary part of development, especially during puberty.

3. Practice taking people, especially females, seriously for what they say, feel, and do, not for how they look.

4. Scrutinize your child's school for things (posters, books, contest) which endorse the cultural ideal of thinness. Watch also for the failure of the school to include images of successful females in the curriculum. Without such images, girls are left with media definitions of thinness as a primary means of success for females.

5. Encourage children to ignore body shape as an indicator of anything about personality or value. Phrases like "fat slob," "pig out," and "thunder thighs" should be discouraged. It is noteworthy that being teased about body shape is associated with disturbed attitudes about eating.

6. Help your child develop interests and skills which will lead to success, personal expression, and fulfillment without emphasis on appearance.

7. Teach children (a) the dangers of trying to alter body shape through dieting; (b) the value of moderate exercise for health, strength, and stamina; and (c) the importance of eating a variety of nutritious foods. Avoid dichotomizing foods into "good/safe/lowfat vs bad/dangerous/fattening."

8. Encourage your children to be active and to enjoy what their bodies can do and feel like. Do not put your child on a diet or exercise program unless a physician has verified that there truly are medical concerns associated with the child's weight

(which is not very likely).

9. Limit how much television children watch. At least occasionally, watch with them and discuss the images of females presented. Do the same with fashion magazines.

10. Make family meals relaxed and friendly. Refrain from commenting on children's eating, resolving family conflicts at the table, and using food as either punishment or reward.

What men can do

by Michael P. Levine

Men have a special role in helping prevent eating disorders:

● **Take your role as a father, brother and/or uncle seriously.** Men play a very significant role in the emotional and psychosocial development of girls and boys. Abnegation of the role of father, in particular, in the name of work or success or lack of time is a contribution to (a) the emotional distress ("hunger") underlying eating disorders in females; and (b) feelings of powerlessness, insecurity and rage in males that fuel the oppression of women through objectification, pornography and other forms of violence.

● **Take personal and political action against sexism.** Men can contribute to the prevention of eating disorders by changing their own behavior and/or the behavior of others so as to:
(a) reverse discrimination against girls and women in school, in the workplace, on the streets, and at home;
(b) ensure that girls/women are free from harassment, sexual abuse, physical intimidation and other forms of violence to their bodies and souls;
(c) encourage girls/women (and boys/men) to accept and develop themselves as people, not as attractive packages based on restrictive ideals of beauty and self-restraint;
(d) develop relationships between (and images of) boys/men and girls/women based on respect, not exploitation.[2]

Reprinted with permission from the National Eating Disorders Organization.

NEDO NEWSLETTER, 1994/AFRAID TO EAT 1997

Eating disorders prevention

by Sue Chaussee

1. Build on positives rather than focus on weakness.
2. Provide success experiences.
3. Train in small steps, without embarrassment.
4. Avoid judgments.
5. Teach positive self talk, not negative putdowns.
6. Relabel — find the positive in negatives.
7. Give congruent messages. Avoid sarcasm and watch nonverbal messages.
8. Give affirmations; being is important.
9. Parents are role models — "Children live what they learn."
10. Teach praise. Parents must first praise themselves. Parents must teach children to praise themselves. Parents must praise children for praising themselves and praising others.
11. Pay attention to good behavior.
12. Talk with kids about their positives.
13. Talk with kids about media myths. Such as smiling women scrubbing toilet bowls, skinny people eating chips and drinking beer, and winners wearing special athletic shoes.
14. Beware of cultural myths about men and women and their value. Don't contribute to the myth that a woman's appearance determines her value.
15. Encourage and support friendships outside the family.
16. Eat in healthy ways.
17. Avoid restricting food, fad diets or dieting — this encourages weight gain and/or development of eating disorders.
18. Do not pressure family members for thinness.
19. Teach family members to express all their feelings at appropriate level for developmental stage. Role model emotional expression also — most women have the most difficulty expressing anger.
20. Make meal times pleasant and fun.[3]

SUE CHAUSSEE, LSW, 1992. ARCHWAY FAMILY SERVICES, BISMARCK, ND/AFRAID TO EAT 1997

Parents may want to examine their own feelings about weight and food, and work toward self-acceptance and size-acceptance. Modeling healthy behavior means having ordinary nondiet foods and meals in the home, and exercising for fun and fitness, not appearance.

Once the child is in treatment, the helpful parent will be there to listen, keeping communication open, and sharing in supportive ways, says Fortin. Parents may wonder whether they are too involved or not involved enough. They need to allow their eating-disordered teen to grow up, to do the things others her age are doing. Giving advice and opinions in a respectful manner, as they would with another adult, will help.

But parents are not responsible for making the eating disordered patient well, she cautions. "The therapist will be responsible for that portion of the recovery process. This does not mean that you ignore the eating disorder altogether: Your support is important."

The therapist can help parents with coping strategies. Don't let the eating disorder take over all of family life, Fortin advises. Focus on other interests you share. If family communication has broken down, family therapy may be advised. Recovery may be slow, and parents should not be discouraged by good progress followed by a plateau or setback. This is part of normal recovery. This is hard work, so families can celebrate small improvements.

Fortin offers these tips for parents of eating disordered youth:

■ Learn as much as you can about eating disorders. You can be supportive by just understanding the issues your teen will be facing in therapy.

■ Focus on issues of health and well-being. Avoid commenting on the person's weight or appearance. She/he is already overly focused on it.

■ Understand the eating behavior as a problematic coping strategy for dealing with painful emotions and conflicts. Do not blame or shame the person.

■ Encourage discussion around the person's current conflicts and concerns. Be prepared to help problem-solve and find supportive help from a professional.

- Be prepared to seek help and support for the entire family. This is a good way to develop mutually respectful coping strategies.

- Youth with eating disorders may benefit from structure and consistency in family meals. Regard meals as an opportunity for a relaxed time during which family members can catch up with each other's interests. Do not put undue focus on food, or force or withhold food.

- Avoid power struggles over food. Do not prepare or buy food for the adolescent and other food for the rest of the family.

- When the behavior of the eating disordered person affects others, she/he is responsible. Bathrooms and kitchens should be left clean by everyone. Household or shared foods depleted by bingeing should be replaced by the person who binged.

- Take the adolescent to your doctor for medical evaluation if you are at all worried about her physical status. Signs of medical instability can be subtle, and might include dizziness, tingling sensations and "blacking out."

Helping the large child

It is time to look at childhood obesity in different ways.

Most parents are very aware of the social stigma associated with being fat. Many of them have experienced size discrimination first hand, and all of them have witnessed it. They are determined not to let this happen to their children. But the steps they take to prevent obesity may backfire.

When parents are afraid that a child is becoming fat, they often restrict food, says Joanne Ikeda. But recent research shows this can backfire. Children whose parents control their food intake show less ability to self-regulate energy intake. As a consequence, they may be at higher risk of obesity than children who are allowed to choose how much food they consume.[6]

Therapists often find these children beg, scavenge, and even steal food because of their fear of hunger. Some parents act more like

Guidelines for approaching a person with an eating disorder

General guidelines

● Recognize your own attitude and amount of focus on your weight, body shape, and dieting practices. How might this be triggering or encouraging a friend, family member, or child to follow your pattern?

● Try not to use food as a socializing agent.

● Recognize that food has a purpose: to fulfill hunger.

● If there are family or friendship disagreements, try not to argue at the table. Such negative experiences become associated with eating and then food is thought of as a problem.

● Allow the eating disordered person to be in charge of their own eating.

● Avoid monitoring the food that the person eats, once the person is in treatment.

Guidelines for family members and friends

● Do not treat the person with an eating disorder like a child. If you are a parent, do not deny your daughter or son some parental guidance, but at the same time remember that he/she has many adult abilities which need to develop.

● When you speak to the person, speak with compassion and concern. Be as descriptive as possible.

● Avoid focusing on how the person looks with comments such as; "You're looking far too thin," or, "You're looking great!" This encourages body image obsessions. Instead focus on other areas of the person's life as much as possible.

● Explain what you suspect by describing the person's problematic behaviors. State your observations.

● Negotiate acceptable behavior with the person.

● Do not allow the dysfunctional behavior to be overlooked, otherwise, you are rewarding it. You need to increase the person's responsibility for his/her behavior.

● Set rules with the person regarding what is acceptable food to eat and how many meals a day are acceptable. Then focus conversations on other topics.

- If a person is binge eating, discuss with the person how you could help him/her.

- Do not use scare tactics. They are not appropriate and do not work.

- Give the person time to improve unless you suspect that his/her life is in danger. Negotiate a plan that may include certain behaviors such as eating regularly or decreasing purging. If the verbal contract is broken, seek professional help.

- If a person appears to be showing signs of extreme physical problems yet refuses help, a decision needs to be made by the parents and professionals to determine if treatment is necessary and how to initiate it.

- Try not to spy or interfere once the person with an eating disorder is in treatment.

- Provide specific information for help; names of treatment providers, phone numbers. There may be eating disorder specialists in your community or there may be support groups for eating disorders. Have the information available when you approach the person.

Guidelines regarding the person with an eating disorder

- The person with an eating disorder is sensitive to nonverbal behavior judging others' attitudes toward them by a fleeting expression, a tone of voice, or even the movement of your body.

- Try to remember their intense feelings of inadequacy. Attitudes of scorn, disgust, or impatience exhibited toward a person with an eating disorder intensifies his/her symptoms.

- Recognize that the person may deny your observations and be upset (especially if anorexic). Try not to be discouraged. Recognize that you have broken through his/her psychological defense. The person is frightened.

- Do not expect an immediate 100 percent recovery. As with any disorder, there will be a period of convalescence. There may be relapses. There will be difficult days when all of the old tensions flare up again.[4]

REPRINTED WITH PERMISSION FROM THE NATIONAL EATING DISORDERS ORGANIZATION/
AFRAID TO EAT 1997

prison guards than nurturers and caregivers. Ikeda suggests that health professionals must assure parents that infants are born with the ability to regulate their own energy intake and that this ability needs to be fostered, rather than interfered with.

Even if we don't actively discriminate against people who deviate too greatly from our standards for beauty, our silence condones it. Our children watch us and model their behavior after ours.

"Fat has become the bogeyman, the monster that terrorizes our children," Ikeda says. "Overdramatic? Only as dramatic as the newspaper headlines, 'Too Fat Boy Murders Classmates who Teased him, Then Kills Self,' 'Girl drops Dead of Starvation — Afraid of Becoming too Fat,' and 'Girl Commits Suicide because Mom nagged her to Lose Weight.' These are not from the *National Enquirer*. They are all articles I have clipped from California newspapers over the past couple of years."

Ellyn Satter charges that our current attitudes and approaches blame children and parents for a child's fatness and promise cures that health professionals can't deliver.

"We have led parents to believe that children are too fat because they eat too much and that children can become slim if they eat less. In so doing we set parents and children up for disappointment and unnecessary self blame. We have done the same to ourselves. In encouraging patients to try for weight loss, we find ourselves administering programs we don't totally believe in and accepting outcomes that leave us feeling discouraged and dishonest. It's time to define the problem of juvenile obesity in a way it can be solved."

She says we have overreacted to normal fatness and the growth process, which often means children will slim down. However, some children are genetically fat. "It is possible that our interventions — restriction of food intake and subsequent struggles and preoccupation with eating — have exacerbated tendencies to fatness and interfered with a child's normal inclination to slim down. Even when obesity does exist, we don't know what causes it. Fat children eat no more, or no differently, than thin children. Nor do we know how to cure it."

Satter cites research that shows children are less able to regulate how much they eat when parents are preoccupied with keeping them

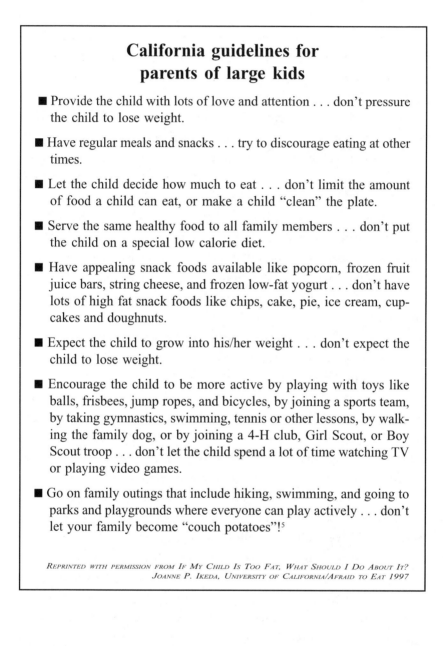

California guidelines for parents of large kids

■ Provide the child with lots of love and attention . . . don't pressure the child to lose weight.

■ Have regular meals and snacks . . . try to discourage eating at other times.

■ Let the child decide how much to eat . . . don't limit the amount of food a child can eat, or make a child "clean" the plate.

■ Serve the same healthy food to all family members . . . don't put the child on a special low calorie diet.

■ Have appealing snack foods available like popcorn, frozen fruit juice bars, string cheese, and frozen low-fat yogurt . . . don't have lots of high fat snack foods like chips, cake, pie, ice cream, cupcakes and doughnuts.

■ Expect the child to grow into his/her weight . . . don't expect the child to lose weight.

■ Encourage the child to be more active by playing with toys like balls, frisbees, jump ropes, and bicycles, by joining a sports team, by taking gymnastics, swimming, tennis or other lessons, by walking the family dog, or by joining a 4-H club, Girl Scout, or Boy Scout troop . . . don't let the child spend a lot of time watching TV or playing video games.

■ Go on family outings that include hiking, swimming, and going to parks and playgrounds where everyone can play actively . . . don't let your family become "couch potatoes"![5]

REPRINTED WITH PERMISSION FROM IF MY CHILD IS TOO FAT, WHAT SHOULD I DO ABOUT IT? JOANNE P. IKEDA, UNIVERSITY OF CALIFORNIA/AFRAID TO EAT 1997

from being fat.[7] She says when parents restrain food and fail to gratify children's appetites, they can lose their ability to regulate food and when controls are relaxed are prone to overeat. She reports that children can get too fat when they are systematically overfed, although normally if overfed, the child will compensate by eating less the next day.[8]

They can get too fat when their emotional needs are not met, when they don't feel safe, when there is stress in the family or the environment. Among typical responses to these situations, children may overdemand food as a way of attracting the parents' attention or become underactive because they are despondent. A child may also overeat because she is depressed or anxious and has learned to use food as a way of soothing her feelings. A child may under exercise because someone is overprotective, is intolerant of her noise and mess, or because she is depressed and lacks the energy to be active.[9]

Satter warns, "In all cases, rather than attempting to shift calorie balance with diet and exercise, it is essential to identify and resolve underlying causes in order to restore the child's normal regulatory and growth patterns. That outcome goal is achievement of the child's weight, not some externally defined (even modest) standard of weight. Striving for a particular body weight creates distortions with eating and feeding and interferes markedly with nurturing the child."

In treatment programs, Satter suggests setting aside weight loss as an outcome goal and focusing instead on achievable goals: treating the attitudes and behaviors that accompany the obesity. "We can help our patients learn to eat and exercise in a healthful and positive way, to feel better about themselves, and to feel good about their bodies. If we — and they — institute these changes, they might be thinner. But we can't count on it, and we must not promise it."

Rather than requiring the child to eat less or exercise more, Satter says the destabilizing influences must be identified and corrected to restore the child's normal regulatory and growth processes.

Helping parents understand feeding management may correct the underlying cause of a child's energy imbalance, but it must be focused on parents' feeding practices rather than on what and how much children eat, she says.

"Positive feeding demands a division of responsibility: Parents need to be primarily responsible for planning and procuring the family food supply, for maintaining the structure of meals and snacks and for limiting between-meal panhandling," says Satter.

"Given a feeding environment that is pleasant, supportive, and

Intervening with childhood obesity

Maintain structured meals and snacks

- Have meals and snacks at reliable times
- Limit *random* eating and (caloric) drinking between times

Maintain a division of responsibility in feeding

- Parents take primary responsibility for planning, procuring, preparing
- Let *even the fat child* decide what and how much to eat from what has been provided
- Don't criticize how much the child eats or give the child "looks."

Help the child to detect and trust hunger, appetite and satiety

- Have pleasant eating times where the child can be relaxed
- Teach and model focused, mindful eating
- Expect reasonably civilized table manners — be realistic
- Don't promote "stocking up" sometimes by restricting food other times
- Don't reward with food or use it for comfort — but do be supportive

Cut down on feeding cues (reminders)

- Confine most eating to the table
- Make most eating at either meal or snack time
- Put food out of sight to limit absent-minded eating
- Turn off the TV at eating times.

Keep the caloric density of food moderate

- Make moderate use of high-fat, high-sugar foods
- Don't deprive the child of such "treat" foods: that makes them more appealing

Think of the child as "normal" when making food decisions

- Plan and provide nutritious meals and snacks
- Make food selection decisions as you would for any child
- Trust your child's food regulation — don't fake it by serving low-calorie food

Use your own good judgment in setting feeding limits

- It is helpful to teach orderly, deliberate and satisfying eating
- It is helpful to be firm about structure with eating

- It is not helpful to deprive

Look for causes if a child's growth changes

- Children's growth is ordinarily stable — if it changes, there has to be a reason

Goals in treatment programs

- Be realistic about outcome
- Allow the child to develop the weight that's right for him/her
- Maintain a positive feeding relationship — parent and child *share* responsibility for eating
- Prevent overeating. (*Don't* promote undereating)
- Develop regular and reasonable exercise
- Support/enhance social functioning, including coping with a "handicapping condition"[6]

allows them the freedom to pick and choose from food that the parent has made available, children can take responsibility for deciding what and how much they will eat. It is when parents don't execute their feeding responsibilities or intrude on the child's prerogatives that feeding difficulties and disturbances of food regulation occur. Parents may fail to get a meal on the table, then try to control what and how much their child eats."

However, Satter finds that some parents are so rigid and controlling, or so fearful of the child's obesity, that they can't trust the child in the area of eating. Other parents are so chaotic, both internally and externally, that they can't bring order into feeding. At both extremes, families require referral to mental health professionals to correct the rigidity and/or chaos.

Frequently, these families will not participate in treatment and only want the child to be put on a diet. Such efforts should be avoided. "It is absolutely unrealistic to expect the child to lose weight when the whole family system is set up to promote the opposite."

Putting a child on a weight reduction diet, or restricting food intake in even indirect ways (such as specifying "free" and "limited" foods) profoundly distorts the developmental needs of both parents and children. Children need to be nurtured. Parents need to nurture. Children need to be able to trust their internal processes. Parents need to be able to relax and trust their children and those processes — not be police officers.

For children who are genetically obese (or who remain obese despite restoration of positive feeding and family dynamics), additional treatment strategies are in order. The goal for this child is to allow her to grow up to achieve a healthy body and feel good about that body and about herself.

Fat children can be physically active and successful in certain sports. Fat children can feel good about their eating, and have varied diets of high nutritional quality. And fat children can have good social and emotional skills. In fact, to be successful, fat children must acquire better-than-average social and emotional skills, says Satter.

Obesity is a stigmatizing condition. Children who grow up with this condition, and their parents, need help learning to deal with the prejudice and social and emotional challenges obesity presents. Fat children grow up to think less of themselves only if their parents think less of them. Some parents are unaccepting and vehement about trying to change their children. Others blame themselves for their child's condition and are overprotective.

Fat children grow up to feel good about themselves if their families value them for their considerable worth, expect them to be capable, and see the obesity as only one of a range of characteristics.[10]

Prevention starts at birth

To the extent that it is an abnormal and unnecessary condition for the child, obesity can be prevented, Satter explains. This process starts at birth, with a positive feeding relationship between parent and child. Infants know how much they need to eat. They give cues to guide the feeding process, and to grow properly they must be supported in eating according to their internal regulatory processes of hunger, appetite and satiety.

For the parents of the obese child, an important part of prevention is helping them resist pressure to put their child on a weight reduction diet. Parents feel guilty and responsible when a child is too fat.

Their guilt is reinforced by health professionals, school, media, family and friends who think parents have "done something wrong" and expect them to remedy it. Parents don't benefit from criticism. They need help with their feelings, and support in pursuing a moderate approach.

Weight may level off and allow a child to rejoin an earlier, lower weight curve. However, trying for this outcome amounts to an attempt at weight loss that will distort the feeding relationship, Satter warns. Rather than trying for weight loss, we must measure outcome by the degree to which we have helped the parents and child establish positive eating and exercise behavior and functional social and emotional skills. Then we must let weight find its own level.

Of course, we can continue to hope that if families achieve these goals, children will grow up to be slim — or at least slimmer than they would be otherwise. The odds are good: Longitudinal studies show us that more children slim down than stay fat. We can help children institute positive lifelong eating and exercise patterns and attitudes toward self and others. We can let them grow up to get the bodies that are right for them. But we can't make them lose weight. We can only do all we can — then we must let go of it.[11]

Joanne Ikeda conducted weight management programs in the early 1980s for teens using a behavior modification approach.[12,13]

"Some of the youngsters I worked with lost weight, some maintained, and some gained," she reports. "All of them needed more love and acceptance. There was the large boned, aristocratic looking girl accompanied by a mother who wore a size four petite. 'I hope you can do something with her, because I can't,' said the mother haughtily. I felt like saying, 'Sure, I'll just touch her with my magic wand and make her look just like you,' but of course, I didn't.

"There were two bosom buddies; one looked fatter than the other. The larger girl kept worrying that her friend would lose weight, and thus have no need of their friendship. She made sure they visited the candy machine before and after every meeting.

"The only adolescent who appeared to have escaped serious damage to his self-esteem was a big kid whose mother brought him in, saying, 'Everyone in our family is big, so I don't expect him to lose weight. I just want him to learn some healthy habits.'

"'Yes, yes, yes!' was my enthusiastic response. She was right, this boy was big. Big enough to intimidate any peers who wanted to make his size an issue. Plus he was good at using humor to help our group 'lighten up,' and even I was vulnerable to his charm. We needed his levity to ease the pain — the pain of knowing that your parents would love you more, your teachers would like you more, and your life would be wonderful if you could just look like the kids featured in *Sassy, Seventeen,* or *Young and Modern.*

"I stopped working with fat youngsters when I realized that I was contributing to their distress by reinforcing the idea that there was something 'wrong' with their bodies. But their pain remains with me. It sustains me and provides the motivation for my efforts to promote size acceptance in some very concrete ways."

Children have no control over their genetic make-up, and health professionals need to help parents be realistic, Ikeda points out. "When a tall, large man and a short, fragile-looking woman have children, they may expect their daughters to resemble the mother, and sons, the father. But this may not be the case."

Parents who try to pressure children by making their love conditional on weight loss, need to be told that they are harming, not helping, their children, she says. Size discrimination is often practiced under the guise that it will motivate large children to change their eating and exercise habits so their bodies will become "normal."

Health care professionals are in a unique position to influence attitudes and opinions, and point out flaws in this thinking.

"Our children did not create this world where an overabundance of appealing, low-cost, high-fat foods are widely available at a moment's notice. A world where machines perform most of the tasks that used to require human energy expenditure. As adults, we must assume the responsibility for this situation and make every effort to change it. The problems are ours to deal with in ways that help, not punish our children."[14,15]

Raising largely positive kids

Big kids have a hard time in our thin-obsessed society.

Carol Johnson, author of *Self-Esteem Comes in All Sizes,* and founder of Largely Positive support groups, says adults must send them enough positive, loving messages to counteract the negative ones they'll hear at school, the beach, at parties, and from the media.

"As hard as it is to be a fat adult in America, it's even harder for fat kids. Kids long to fit in and be accepted by their peers. Damage to self-esteem can begin at a very young age. If it's not mended, the scars can last a lifetime.

"I'm not opposed to weight loss. What troubles me is our inability to separate weight loss from self-esteem. Large kids should not be led to believe losing weight will make them better people. Because despite their best efforts, not all kids will lose weight permanently.

"It's imperative that parents and supportive adults provide larger kids with the tools to realize they're just as good as thinner kids, that weight is not a measure of their self-worth."

Johnson's suggestions for raising largely positive kids are:

■ Be sure your understanding of obesity is accurate and that you can separate myths from facts. This will help you to view a child's chubbiness as physiology, rather than a "defect."

■ Do *not* put a larger child on a diet. Most experts now agree this is one of the worst things done to overweight children.

■ Teach larger children that their self-worth has nothing to do with their weight. Emphasize their positive attributes and talents, and teach them that these are the things that have lasting value. Give frequent praise for talents, accomplishments and for just being who they are.

■ Be honest with larger children about remarks they are apt to encounter about their weight. Help them decide how they will respond. Tell them that many groups of people have suffered discrimination, and that larger people are one of those groups. Teach them that diversity of size is no different from diversity of culture — we must learn to respect both.

■ Be a good role model. Don't criticize your own body. If children see you appreciate your own body, they'll find it easier to like themselves.

■ Don't *ever* suggest that a larger child's weight makes him/her less attractive or that no one will want to date them. This can cause lifelong damage to self-esteem. In a similar vein, teach them to respect themselves. A larger young girl may be thankful for any attention a boy gives her. Teach her that she deserves respect and affection and that anything less should not be tolerated.

■ Make an extra effort to help your larger child find clothes that are in style.

■ Encourage physical activity. But let the child decide what activities he or she prefers. Don't force a larger little girl into a ballet class if she doesn't feel comfortable there. On the other hand, if she wants to twirl a baton, don't discourage her because of her size. Physical activity can be a family affair. Take a family walk every evening or set up a badminton game. When I was a young adult, I went jogging with my dad. It was a nice time for both of us.[16,17]

Children need reassurance that human beings come in a wide variety of sizes and shapes, and that there is no "ideal" or "perfect" body. They should be taught that every body is a good body, and that each person is responsible for taking care of his or her body. Most importantly, children should learn to respect the bodies of others even when they are quite different from their own.

CHAPTER 11

Prevention in schools

■

Schools reflect society's obsession with thinness and scorn for large people. The pressure, the harassment is all there — between students, between teachers, in the classrooms and in the halls.

Teachers tell me that they see girl after girl in the lunchroom choosing the salad bar over main-course meals, and coming out with only a small plate of lettuce. "I hope they are making up for it with healthy meals at home," one teacher said. Then she sighed — we both knew it wasn't happening at home, either.

This mini-world is an important and natural player in the effort for change. But a greater awareness is needed so parents and educators will recognize eating and weight problems, and decide to approach them in a comprehensive way using new paradigm concepts which benefit all children and harm none.

Schools have long recognized the problem of hungry children. Many provide lunch and breakfast for kids who are neglected, low income, or whose parents both work.

This is just one step. It does not begin to touch the problems of girls and boys hungry from self-starvation. Schools could do far more to address the role they play in children's lives when it comes to eating, socializing and developing self respect — qualities that aren't part of the curriculum but are nonetheless part of the learning process.

"A student who is not healthy, who suffers from an undetected vision or hearing defect, or who is hungry, or who is impaired by drugs or alcohol, is not a student who will profit from the educational process," says Michael McGinnis, director of the Office of Disease Prevention and Health Promotion.[1]

Today one in four children lives with a single parent; one in five lives in poverty; one in five is of a minority race; and one in 10 has a physical or mental disability, factors which may increase the risk of health problems and educational failure, says Lloyd J. Kolbe, PhD, Chief, Office of School Health and Special Projects, Centers for Disease Control, Atlanta. The major health problems our society faces are caused in large part by behaviors begun during youth, he notes.

Given these challenges, school health programs can become one of the most efficient means the nation could employ to prevent the major health problems that confront us, he says. Comprehensive school health programs can prevent future health problems, improve economic productivity, reduce the spiraling costs of health care, and improve educational outcomes. Schools can prevent many health problems from happening, detect others at early stages, and treat those that have not been prevented, thus avoiding the worst effects. Kolbe calls for a regeneration of school health programs to bring about these changes.[2]

An awareness of the severity of the weight and eating crisis for youth today and effective preventive measures fit well into this scenario.

Unifying the approach

Most schools use the Comprehensive School Health Program, a new unified approach, developed by Kolbe and the Centers for Disease Control and Prevention Division of Adolescent School Health. This program recognizes that education and health are interrelated and that healthy children who feel safe and accepted in their environment can learn better and achieve more academically.

Comprehensive school health programs provide unique opportunities throughout the school experience for health promotion and preventive health measures. They make important changes in the health and lives of the 45 million American youth who attend school every school day, and for their families, the school staff and community.

The CDC program includes the following eight interdependent components, all important in a comprehensive school program that addresses eating and weight issues:

■ Health education
■ Physical education and activity
■ Counseling services
■ Food service
■ Healthy school environment
■ Health programs for faculty and staff
■ Health services
■ Parent and community involvement

In each of these eight components, schools address six high risk behaviors: injuries from accidents, violence, suicide; tobacco use; alcohol and other drug use; poor nutrition; lack of physical activity; and sexual behavior, sexually transmitted diseases and HIV, and unwanted pregnancies.

Many of these risky behaviors are involved with body image, weight and eating. Poor nutrition and lack of physical activity are closely related to a wide range of eating and weight problems. Violence, harassment and suicide are linked to dysfunctional eating, eating disorders and related low self-esteem and depression. Sexual or physical abuse often appears to trigger eating disorders. Teenage girls smoke to lose weight and won't quit for fear of weight gain. And the risk of preteen pregnancies increases with early puberty, apparently related to higher levels of body fat and sedentary living.

The challenge is to develop and integrate into the school's health program the components that can prevent obesity, eating disorders, dysfunctional eating and size prejudice. Such a program will not only diminish weight and eating problems, but also reduce the health problems, permanent injury and deaths caused by weight loss efforts. It can do much to stimulate students' intellectual growth and their ability to learn.

Health education

In the classroom, health education can help youngsters integrate normal eating, healthy food choices, and balanced, active living from kindergarten through high school. Classroom curriculums can expand to deal with the level of eating disorders, dysfunctional eating, overweight and size prejudice that are real issues for students today. Creating awareness is a first step to help teachers recognize eating problems, dangerous weight loss practices, and size oppression so they can be dealt with at early stages.

At junior high and high school levels, required classes in nutrition, child development and family living give students a solid foundation to incorporate the healthy living and family concepts from these fields into their lives.

Unfortunately, in these days of tight budgets many schools have cut back on these very classes. Parent and community involvement make a big difference in influencing these decisions. Concerned parents who recognize how fundamental these subjects are to healthy living can insist their schools require, or at least offer, these classes and that their own youngsters take them.

The eating and weight crisis is truly a health emergency and we must treat it this way.

Everywhere I go now people tell their terrible stories with haunted eyes: a sister who doesn't eat; a beloved granddaughter, 16, hospitalized in long-term care for her anorexia; a daughter with bulimia who quit college because she couldn't focus her thoughts when taking tests; a nephew's suicide related to his body shame and being picked on in school; a stepdaughter who "lives on coffee and cigarettes."

Teachers are hearing these same stories and watching them being played out every day in their classrooms.

Antismoking programs in schools which are aware of these problems will incorporate information on the relationship of smoking to weight. Bonnie Spring, PhD, of Chicago Medical School, suggests targeting teenage girls with messages about the small effect of smoking on weight-suppression, that minimize excessive concern with weight related to stopping smoking, and emphasize the higher health risks of smoking versus lower risks of weight gain.

Physical education and activity

Healthy kids have daily opportunities to exercise, play and learn new skills in school to help them maintain strong and healthy bodies.

Many schools are well on their way to shifting physical education emphasis toward keeping all youngsters active in ways that last a lifetime. These schools focus more on getting all kids involved, and less on winning games, grooming star athletes and showcasing spectator sports. They don't excuse youngsters with special needs from PE, but broaden programs to include them.

Good things are happening for girls in sports and athletics. In the two decades since Title IX mandated equality for female athletics in schools, the percent of girls in sports has grown from 4 to 42 percent. And 27 percent of high school girls play on sports teams run outside of school. Schools are trying to increase class time and improve the quality of physical education so it provides both training in lifetime skills and the daily exercise needed by today's youngsters, who are often inactive outside school.

Healthy People 2000, which sets the nation's health goals, calls for daily physical education for all students and that 50 percent of class time be spent actively by every child.

Physical education has often focused on helping athletic students become even better. Today it is seen as even more urgent to help physically underdeveloped children, since these are the very youngsters who need activity most and are most likely to lead sedentary lives.

Focusing physical activity on fun and creativity, not competition, is important to these kids. Competition isolates and discourages them from being active. With special help they can keep motivated, and find pleasure and success in physical activity. The President's Council on Physical Fitness and Sports identifies this as "the most urgent task facing physical education and other youth programs." The Council recommends fitness testing and remedial programs for students who don't meet standards. But sensitivity is important, as are new ways to avoid stigmatizing or humiliating the less fit and larger youngsters.

Additionally, many experts are calling for more after school in-tramural sports, shifting the focus of the school's resources away from training a winning team. More kids get to play on intramural teams. Communities that support intramural sports find it can be difficult to compete for time, gymnasiums and coaching staff, but that children in intramural sports often have more fun and it lessens the sometimes-bitter competition between schools. Dedicated ath-letes, too, can benefit from a more open system that frees up their time for other interests.

Counseling services

School counselors help identify factors that hinder optimum school performance and adjustment, provide broad-based intervention pro-grams, and connect students to appropriate services. Integration of weight and eating issues into the counseling program is important in helping schools deal effectively with related problems. School coun-selors need special training in nutrition, weight and eating issues. Or a staff nutritionist who is a family and consumer teacher, home econo-mist or nutrition specialist can help in this role.

Ideally, school districts will staff nutrition counselors or nutrition teachers to help students and train teachers in weight and eating issues. This is a major health crisis, and school administrators, boards and parents need to take effective steps to address these problems.

The counselor may form support groups for students with prob-lem eating and weight issues, refer students to specialists when needed, and work with a team of faculty, parents and community leaders to integrate preventive programs in school, community and the home.

In the role of teacher training, the counselor will increase aware-ness and help them learn to identify potential problems in students. They will also help teachers, staff, coaches and athletic trainers probe their own biases and confront the reality that they may be caught up themselves in the same harmful behaviors as their students with dys-functional eating, muscle building obsessions, body image and size bias.

Assigning a sports nutritionist to work with school athletic teams will also help prevent many problems, such as the dangerous weight loss practices common for athletes in sports like wrestling, gymnastics and running. The counselor or sports nutritionist meets with athletes, coaches and parents at the beginning of each season, and is available for consultation. She helps coaches identify and alleviate obsessive exercise behaviors and disordered eating patterns.

Food service

Nutritious and appealing meals that coordinate with other health and nutrition education help students develop strong healthy bodies and good eating habits. A nutritionist on staff can oversee lunch and breakfast menus and the stocking of vending machines with nutritious food selections, finding creative ways to encourage kids to make healthy food choices and practice healthy eating habits.

Healthy school environment

The goal must be zero tolerance for size bias in the schools, in hallways, grounds and classrooms.

Physical, emotional and social surroundings which are safe, secure and accepting of each individual will enhance the well being, intellectual development, and productivity of students and staff. If kids feel safe they are freer to direct energies to learning and can develop in natural, healthful ways. Victims will be liberated.

Size prejudice not only hurts large kids but all kids, because it warns them they can never be thin enough. It keeps all kids striving to be thinner, in their fear of ridicule and rejection. The same fears and biases are reflected by teachers and staff.

With the new recommendations from the National Education Association on combatting size prejudice, now is the ideal time for schools to move ahead with providing an unbiased environment that respects all individuals of all sizes.

In the same way schools are calling for "zero tolerance" for drugs and tobacco, they can establish "zero tolerance for size bias." They can refuse to allow size discrimination, harassment, bullying, or the singling out of any student for special torment.

Administrators and staff have the responsibility of supervising student conduct and protecting students. School policies and how they are carried out give students important guidelines in learning how to get along in society. Children will perform according to the expectations their teachers have of them. And insisting on respect for each individual and encouraging self respect does work.

In many schools, creating awareness programs for teachers and staff will be a first step. Teachers may need to assess their own attitudes and behaviors about weight so they don't inadvertently model body dissatisfaction or promote size discrimination, suggests Joanne Ikeda, nutrition specialist at the University of Calif., Berkeley. She advises using the National Association to Advance Fat Acceptance self-assessment measure for this purpose.[3]

Other schools may want to begin by surveying potential problems and developing focus groups to study them.

A program to teach students about size bias, reduce size prejudice and the stigmatization of large students has been developed by the Council on Size and Weight Discrimination, led by Nancy Summer, Bearsville, N.Y., and Cathi Rodgveller, of Seattle.[4]

In her workshops for sixth to ninth grade girls, Summer begins by inviting students to "get all the negative things out of their systems that they think and say about fat people . . . 'What do you think when you see a person as fat as me?'" Summer brings out the stereotypes and negative language, writing the words on a flip chart, countering the negative stereotypes with facts and personal stories. She also discusses healthy alternatives to dieting and weight obsession.

"We cover a lot of ground in the workshops: everything from discrimination to health to sports to fashion magazines. But always I stress my basic message: bias against fat hurts people of all sizes . . . I explain that it isn't just large kids and adults who are hurt by size discrimination. Everyone else is hurt, because as long as fat is hated, everyone will be afraid of becoming fat . . . I share a lot of personal stories and listen to theirs. Some of the stories I hear are sad and frightening."

An important part of the workshops is looking at models and classic art, comparing fashion layouts from *Vogue* and *Big Beautiful Woman,* and discussing the difference between glamour and thinness. Summer says the girls usually tell her the larger models are the prettiest, "And I have to remind them that girls and women of all sizes are beautiful."

She encourages kids of all sizes to fight size bias by speaking up every time they see it, explaining that fat kids need allies when they are being picked on. They discuss ways of doing this. "It isn't enough to just not laugh along with a joke. It's important that you say something, whether it's privately to the person being picked on, or publicly to the mean kids that what they are doing isn't okay."

This leads to the concept of peer support in dealing with harassments. The bully who yells across the cafeteria, "Hey Fatso!" doesn't just hurt the fat kid, Summer points out. He hurts every boy and girl who hears it. He makes everyone afraid of being picked on. He makes other fat kids afraid they'll be next, and he makes thin kids afraid of getting fat. The possibilities of how students can defend themselves and each other against prejudiced attitudes are explored.

The bully needs to be stopped so that all kids are free to be themselves. By the end of the workshop, the kids really understand this concept, she says.

For the larger girls in the workshops, it is often what they hear their friends and classmates say about how to fight size bias that matter most to them. Summer feels validated by responses such as these:

"I learned that it's not OK to pick on fat kids."

"I learned that I'm okay and that I can be pretty even though I'm fat."

"I learned that my father is okay and that his brothers shouldn't be mean to him. Please send me something I could show my father about this."

An improvisational theater team of high school students in Spearfish, S.D., performs a size prejudice skit in elementary classrooms. They set the scene in a hallway lined with students, through which sixth-grader Josh must walk as classmates point, laugh and ridicule his size. Embarrassed and humiliated, Josh mutters the last line, "I hate this place!"

Then the actors freeze and "processing" begins, led by faculty advisor Sandy Klarenbeek. She asks questions of the audience, and they in turn question the actors, who stay in character: *Who are these kids? What did you see happen? How does it make you feel? Could this happen in your school? How does this feel to you, Josh? How long has this been going on? Is there anyone you can go to for help? Can you think of others who might help you?*

"I try to point out things about Josh that no one knows such as he has his own Harlem bike, he wrestles . . . It is important for them to realize there is more to Josh than his size. He has feelings, and is an individual," says Klarenbeek. "This kind of peer teaching is very effective."

Health programs for faculty and staff

Teachers and staff with healthy lifestyles and attitudes are powerful role models for kids. And since teachers reflect the problems and biases of our society, many will need help with their own weight and eating issues. Thus, there is an urgent need for effective programs for both staff and students.

Health services

The school nurse, public health nurse, and other school resources provide support and a consistent approach with weight and eating issues. They may be involved in testing, identifying students with special needs, and making referrals to health professionals.

Parent and community involvement

Successful programs integrate parents and other community members into school planning and programs. They serve on teams, committees and school health advisory committees and are involved in health conferences, training sessions, and as classroom volunteers.

Moving ahead to integrate school and community efforts, the administrators, teachers, counselors, parents and community leaders, can find ways of extending healthy weight and eating programs into the wider community. To be most effective, school health efforts will be supported and reinforced in the home and throughout the community.

Team conferences

Training conferences and in-service workshops for school staff and community health teams offer excellent opportunities to integrate weight and eating issues into effective programs. Many states bring health teams together for annual training and program planning.

Last summer I had the privilege of presenting awareness seminars at both the North Dakota Roughrider Health Conference and the Wisconsin Wellness Conference. I found teachers deeply concerned about these issues.

Linda Johnson, MS, assistant director of School Health in North Dakota, who organizes the Roughrider conference along with Danielle Kenneweg from the state health department, believes in wellness for the teachers and community members on these teams. Their approach combines personal wellness skills for participants, along with building strong coalition teams and giving them the training and motivation needed to develop school and community health programs.

This approach and the unique collaboration between the two state departments of education and health have made the annual week-long Roughrider Conference a model for other states. Team coalition members include teachers, counselors, administrators, nurses, parents and school board members.

"We in North Dakota consider every teacher a health teacher, both because each is a personal role model and because anyone who reaches into the lives of children has the opportunity to integrate education into all subject areas," explains Johnson.

Teams return home enthusiastic and ready to work on four short-term goals, which further the long-term community action plans they have developed at the conference.

Prevention programs: eating disorders

New preventive programs for weight and eating problems which integrate at least some of the eight components of the CDC program are being pilot tested.

To date, eating disorder prevention programs have produced mixed results; most have proven more effective at increasing knowledge than changing attitudes and behavior.

An intervention which did make a difference at a Toronto ballet school is described by Niva Piran, PhD, of the Ontario Institute for Studies in Education. It was begun because of concern at the high rate of disturbed eating and eating disorders in the school, with nearly two new cases each year of anorexia or bulimia nervosa.[5]

Piran met with all the ballet students, about 100 girls, age 12 to 18, in small focus groups several times a year and used their knowledge and experiences to guide action and systemic changes. Together they created a cycle of dialogue, reflection and action which made changes through a period of eight years. During this eight years of intervention there was just one case of anorexia and one of bulimia. Students who became preoccupied with shape, weight or food issues promptly requested help or were referred by staff for consultation and, if needed, counseling.

The number of graduating students scoring high on eating disorder measures (EAT score) dropped from 48 to 17 percent, and those reporting binge eating dropped from 35 to 13 percent. Surveys showed a decrease in body dissatisfaction, drive for thinness, and dieting and purging patterns. Despite continued pressures for thinness in ballet, these students displayed a healthier approach to their bodies and their eating patterns. Furthermore, they strongly demanded a safe and respectful treatment of their bodies by school staff and peers.

Efforts to stop dysfunctional eating at earlier stages may do much to help prevent eating disorders.

Researchers at the University of Arizona medical school, Linda Estes, PhD, Marjorie Crago, PhD, and Catherine Shisslak, PhD, advise implementing these three levels of prevention efforts:[6]

1. Universal. This approach targets an entire group with a type of intervention considered desirable for everyone.
2. Selective. Aimed at high risk individuals or subgroups.
3. Indicated. Targets individuals with detectable signs or symptoms of disorder, or subclinical eating disorder symptoms.

Prevention costs are lower and success rates higher at early stages than when disturbed eating has progressed to the clinical stage. At that point, patients are difficult to treat, the treatment takes longer, and the disorder is likely to have more severe medical complications.

Estes, Crago and Shisslak are conducting an extensive multi-site study expected to provide information on the progression of disturbed eating, funded by the McKnight Foundation. They will follow girls from fourth through ninth grade over four years, assessing them annually on weight and eating risk factors related to eating disorders. Results will be used to develop programs geared toward the three intervention levels — universal, selective and indicated.

Eating disorders are complex disturbances, often with a history of family enmeshment or traumatic events, and there is debate (especially from the weight loss industry) over whether dieting and the pressures for thinness may be causative factors.

Nevertheless, evidence that at least some girls progress from less to more severe eating problems underscores the importance of recognizing and preventing the whole spectrum of eating disturbances, say the Arizona researchers.

Based on the information she gleaned from focus groups, Piran sees the cultural pressure for thinness as an interrelated factor. "I conceive of it as a form of violation of women's ownership of their bodies and related to other expressions of this theme, such as: harassment, violence, silencing, deprecation or isolation."

Finding ways to stop these violations of self in the home, school and community is of critical importance in reducing eating disorders.

From the school's viewpoint, another compelling reason to stop violence and harassment is that it is against the law and can invite lawsuits. Some states, such as California, have instituted strong policies to deal with sexual harassment in schools.

Issues strong by fifth grade

Many eating disorder specialists now believe eating disorder prevention programs aimed at adolescents come too late. By junior high, negative eating attitudes and behaviors are strongly ingrained, almost a part of female teenage culture, they warn.

Introducing eating disorder prevention programs in high school is definitely too late, says Margo Maine, PhD, Institute of Living, in Hartford, Conn. Studies show these kinds of programs result in increased awareness of signs, symptoms and side effects but do not change behavior. She says it's unfortunate that so much time has been wasted on this effort too late in the process.

Preventive efforts need to begin in middle elementary grades, say Smolak and Levine. By then, their studies show 30 to 50 percent of American girls already "feel too fat" and 20 to 40 percent are dieting. By eighth grade, over 50 percent of girls say they have dieted during the past year. By high school, 40 to 60 percent of girls feel overweight and are trying to lose. Further, these figures do not reflect the immense pressure felt for body dissatisfaction by other girls who are not dieting.[7]

These attitudes and behaviors are measurable in elementary school, they report, but they show younger girls lack the dieting commitment of older girls. Their beliefs about the importance of thinness have not yet crystallized. Smolak and Levine studied dieting attitudes and behavior in grades one through five and found that by fifth grade, body shape is much more important. Therefore, they recommend that until about this age the focus should be on learning about healthy nutrition, positive eating habits and body acceptance, not eating disorders.

What to do in elementary school

Children who are already dieting in elementary school may be at increased risk for developing eating disorders because of the mental and physical effects of calorie restriction and weight loss failures.

Yet their susceptibility to thinness messages may be modifiable at this point. This is a time when children's social attitudes and beliefs can be changed, their thinness attitudes are still evolving, and it is likely that parents can and will prohibit extreme dieting.

Discussion of eating disorders should begin between fourth and sixth grade when puberty development becomes obvious. For girls this is even younger than age eleven, and certainly before junior high, "before their self-esteem begins to plummet for other reasons," says eating disorder specialist Paula Levine.[8]

Yet, eating disorder specialists warn there is risk that giving symptoms of eating disorders too plainly, such as explaining vomiting and laxative use, may unintentionally promote them.

While fourth or fifth grade may be early enough for discussion of eating disorders in schools, it may not be early enough for parents. Paula Levine speaks to parents of newborn infants in newborn classes about eating disorders, and believes this may have an important impact.

Eating disorder prevention programs should have the following goals and principles, say Smolak and Michael Levine.

Goals:

- Acceptance of diverse body shapes. This should include discussion of the causes of body size and shape and prejudice against heavy people, as well as information about body changes in puberty.
- Understanding that body shape is not infinitely mutable.
- Understanding proper nutrition, including the importance of dietary fat and risks of malnutrition.
- Discussion of the negative effects of dieting as well as the lack of long-term positive effects.
- Information on the positive effects of moderate exercise and the negative effects of excessive exercise.
- Development of strategies to resist teasing, pressure to diet, and propaganda about the importance of slenderness.

Principles:

- Involve parents. Parental cooperation is needed to attain program goals. Possible family problems may be averted or improved. They include mothers who are dieting and worried about their own or their daughter's weight, teasing by family members, negative or detrimental parental control over family eating. It is helpful for parents to examine their own values about body fat, dietary fat and attractiveness. Some children diet even to dangerous levels because of parental encouragement.
- Tailor materials to the child's level. Instead of expecting young children to draw conclusions about how they should behave, simple "rules" might be provided, such as "children should play outside for an hour or more daily, and limit television watching." Discussion on dieting might focus on the short-

term effects such as hunger, crankiness, poor concentration and fatigue.

■ Provide new ways to classify, evaluate and interact with people. Relabeling might involve using characteristics ranging from reliability to kindness to assess a person's value. It is especially important for girls to find attributes other than attractiveness or body shape by which to judge themselves and their success, such as academic, personal or social labels.

■ Focus on healthy nutrition and body acceptance. For third grade and younger the prevention programs should probably avoid presenting the symptoms of eating disorders and disordered eating. But parents and school staff need to know the indicators of eating problems and that such disorders can occur in younger children.

In the Seattle area an eating disorders prevention puppet show is making a big hit in elementary schools. Developed by EDAP (Eating Disorders Awareness and Prevention, Inc.) with professional puppeteers, the Early Childhood Prevention Puppets bring an important message into schools: "It's What's Inside that Counts." The shows are presented by a group of volunteers who undergo a series of training sessions.[9]

Eating disorder specialists say it is important to teach students how to evaluate advertising and its influence on the editorial text of magazines. Educate students to be insulated against the messages on thinness in advertising and the media, they urge; encourage them to write letters to advertisers and boycott products which are offensively advertised.

Obesity prevention programs

Obesity experts say that the first priorities for school-based programs aimed at preventing overweight are modifying school lunches and making sure all students take physical education and that PE does its job.

As they address overweight, it is important for teachers to be aware that emphasizing obesity and its risks in preventive programs can easily escalate into promoting fear of fat, thin mania, eating disorders, censure by health-care providers against persons with weight problems, social and economic discrimination, and the proliferation of hazardous weight loss methods.

The risk of intensifying existing problems is even more acute when dealing with the vulnerability of children. The wrong kind of intervention is worse than excess weight, warns Ellyn Satter. She advises that any programs for overweight children need to enhance psychosocial effects and ensure that no child is stigmatized.

The branch of the National Institutes of Health which is charged with implementing the Obesity Education Initiative in schools was expected to target large children for special obesity education and treatment when it convened a major school conference in 1992. But it was soon clear that educators were asking the National Heart, Lung and Blood Institute for a new approach.[10]

Speakers noted that at least half of dieting adolescents are not overweight, and even for large youth, the physiological and psychological hazards of dieting may outweigh the possible benefits.

Educators warned that it is increasingly important for schools and health professionals to provide sound health information and not simply follow traditional thinking. Dieting should not be recommended for adolescents, said one of the presenters, Pauline Powers, MD. Instead, she said there is need for public education programs to emphasize the acceptance of a range of normal body sizes and shapes.

"Food restriction decreases basal metabolic rate, decreases lean body mass and, with the almost inevitable regaining of weight, may increase total fat," she warned.

Members of the group focusing on younger children at this conference expressed much concern about stigmatizing children at high risk for overweight in school prevention programs. If children at high risk are targeted, they warned, it will likely increase chronic dieting and eating disorders, as well as stigmatize large children. They recommended that no child be singled out for special efforts, but that all be targeted for the NHLBI Obesity Education Initiative. They also bluntly expressed their concern that many of the changes specialists at the conference were recommending focused more on restricting diet than increasing physical activity.

"Focus on how to make them healthier, as opposed to thinner, especially because making them thinner often does not make them healthy," they advised.

Similarly, the adolescent study group warned that NIH's national messages on obesity and weight may further stigmatize high-risk adolescents and lead to body image disturbances, eating disorders and decreased self worth. They, too, recommended targeting all youth, not singling out those at high risk.

They further advised evaluating what is being taught on college campuses about the "Freshman 10," or the 10- to 15-pound weight increase commonly experienced during the first year at college. Maybe it's a part of normal maturation and not detrimental, they warned.

Any programs that schools develop to address the problems of weight, eating and self-esteem should be based on self trust, such educators and experts advise. Students can be taught to trust their own body signals and needs. They can be liberated from false and narrow images based on appearance, and taught how to evaluate and combat media stereotypes. They can be helped to take the focus off weight loss, and focus on being healthy at the weight they are. In schools with zero tolerance for size bias, kids will be assured of acceptance, regardless of size, shape or appearance. Programs with this new approach empower and strengthen all youngsters.

Don't rate progress by numbers on a scale, or how much weight kids lose, says Linda Omichinski, a registered dietitian and Canadian leader in the new perspective and nondiet movement. Her preventive program, *Teens & Diets: No Weigh*, is being used worldwide to help empower teens to effectively manage their own eating. It can be used in schools in the classroom, in counseling sessions and support groups for students with dysfunctional eating *(see appendix)*.[11]

"For teens, a self reliant, health promotion model is well suited to the increasing need for independence and self concept building that is a normal developmental task of teenagers on the road to adulthood," says Omichinski.

Nebraska trial

One of the most extensive obesity prevention programs is the two-year nutrition and physical activity trial in third and fifth grades in two Nebraska elementary schools, an intervention and a control school.

Regular classroom teachers taught nutrition in 18 modules over two years. School lunches were modified using "LUNCHPOWER!, Healthy School Lunches" program, and the exercise component was based on Physical Best, an American Alliance for Health, Physical Education, Recreation and Dance program.

Nutrition improvements were considered moderately successful, but the exercise component was less successful.[12]

School lunches were improved and the day's intake of fat and sodium reduced, compared to the control school. The modified lunches, dropping fat from 44 to 28 percent, were well accepted and liked by students. The lunch program was easily adopted within four months.

The biggest obstacles came in physical education as it exists today. Not enough time was spent in class, students were inactive during class, and curriculums devoted to team sports made it difficult to shift to lifetime activities. However, improvements were made in cutting waiting time, and aerobic activities which easily fit into students lifestyles were emphasized. Strength activities promoted lean tissue development. Activities were designed so all youngsters exercised their large muscle groups for 30 minutes, three days a week.

But results showed kids changed less than expected in activity. The Nebraska researchers report that most elementary kids average only 25 minutes per week in scheduled physical activities and watch television 24 to 27 hours a week, suggesting activity levels at home are also low. Modest short-term changes were made during class periods, but the activity did not appear to carry over through the rest of the day. Still, these are difficult factors to measure. Expectations may have been too high for only two years in a narrowly focused program.

Another school program showing promise is the Kansas LEAN School Health Project, implemented in two pilot communities in 1992. This focuses on changing behavior through four components: improving school lunch; integrating a nutrition curriculum; modifying the physical education curriculum to allow for daily noncompetitive physical activity; and development of an active community coalition to support the school program and provide additional support activities in the community. Early reports note that students have come to view fitness as part of their family and community lives, not just a school activity.[13]

SPARK project leader James Sallis reviewed seven school-based cardiovascular risk reduction programs and found some modest changes in body fat. None of the programs made much effort to combine education and environmental change. Most did not include either physical education or school lunch modification or involve parents, and they did not emphasize behavioral skill training. Thus, they were not really comprehensive.[14]

Neither did they measure any detrimental effect on dysfunctional eating or the stigmatization of large students.

Increasing activity

Sports Play and Active Recreation for Kids (SPARK) is an ongoing federally-funded program to research ways to restructure the physical education curriculum for elementary schools. The SPARK program emphasizes fitness activities that can be enjoyed over a lifetime such as swimming, biking, walking and aerobics activities. Kids play frisbee games, jump rope, and take aerobic dance classes.

Fifth grade teacher Julie Harris of the Turtleback Elementary School in Rancho Bernardo, Calif., is enthusiastic about her five years teaching the SPARK program. "More kids are more active and even nonathletic students learn skills and achieve a measure of success."

Important features are:

■ Training and follow-up for teachers. During the first year, Project SPARK trainers take a half-day refresher course every four months and are visited weekly by a consultant.
■ A detailed curriculum of four-week units, each centered around a specific sport. Skills transfer from one sport to the next.

"We want to create a model grade school PE program that will help instill lifelong exercise habits," says Sallis. "Because we want to connect physical activity to the rest of children's lives, there is a weekly class on how to develop activity routines outside the classroom. And it includes homework — just as in math classes."

In 12 schools on the Navajo reservation near Window Rock, Ariz., the SPARK program has helped 1,250 children in third through sixth grade integrate activity with their tribal culture, while spending 30 minutes, three times a week in moderate to vigorous activity. The first 15 minutes is spent on teaching aerobic skills, the second 15 minutes on sports skills. Native dances are taught in the aerobics unit.

Project leaders hope this program will make a difference in the high prevalence of overweight among these children. About 27 percent of Navajo children are overweight, and another 12 percent are severely overweight.

"A sedentary lifestyle, lack of facilities in which to exercise, and a diet high in fat foods coupled with a large number of fast food restaurants on the reservation conspire to make it very difficult for both Navajo children and adults to maintain a healthy weight," says Paul Rosengard, a fitness specialist with the project. He says the aim is to turn the kids on to movement, to find activity fun and exciting. "And I think that modest goal has already been achieved."

The SPARK program has demonstrated that an improved physical education curriculum, combined with well-designed training for physical education specialists and classroom teachers, can substantially increase the amount of physical activity children receive in school and can help ensure that the resulting physical education classes are enjoyable, says the Surgeon General's 1996 Report on Physical Activity and Health.

But Sallis concedes that getting children to be active outside school has been more difficult than expected.[15]

Curbing abuses

For sports in which weight is important for peak performance, it is essential that coaches, parents and athletes keep a healthy perspective. Full nutrition and healthy growth and development for the athlete cannot be compromised.

Wisconsin is a leader in working to resolve wrestling's inherent weight problems. The new program has proven so successful in relieving pressure to cut weight, that it has seen a large increase in student participation and become a model for other states.[16]

Wisconsin and many other states now require a minimum of 7 percent body fat for males, based on skinfold measurements by trained certified measurers. In Wisconsin, if a wrestler's predicted weight is 115 pounds, he will be encouraged to wrestle at 119 pounds, and can wrestle no lower than 112. He cannot wrestle in a weight class for which he would need to lose more than three pounds a week. The growth allowance is reinstated, with two additional pounds allowed on Dec. 25 and one pound, Feb. 1.

Healthy eating practices are expected and actively integrated into the training program. A sports nutritionist works with wrestlers, coaches and parents.

Although reluctant at first, coaches now overwhelmingly support the new program, says Don Herrmann, associate director of the Wisconsin Interscholastic Athletic Association.

"Probably 60 percent of wrestling coaches openly opposed this in the early stages. They said we didn't need it, that skinfold measures aren't accurate enough, and it would bring too much attention to wrestling weight concerns."

But he says there was a dramatic swing in acceptance and after only a short time 97 to 98 percent of coaches favored the new program. Coaches in other sports were soon asking to be included.

CHAPTER 12

Healthy choices

■

Healthy lifestyle choices nourish the mind, body and spirit. They include eating well, living actively, and having a relaxed, positive attitude toward life.

It's important to teach children how to make healthy choices to prevent the weight and eating problems that dampen the spirits of so many kids today.

So how do we create an atmosphere that makes healthy choices for youngsters easy and fun, and the natural way to live? It involves families, teachers, schools, health professionals and communities.

I think the Canadian Vitality program provides an excellent road map: "Feeling good about yourself starts by accepting who you are and how you look. Healthy, good-looking bodies come in a variety of shapes and sizes. A good weight is a healthy weight, not necessarily a low weight, so don't let your self-worth be determined by the bathroom scales. Think positive thoughts. Laugh a lot. Spend some time with people who have a positive attitude — the type who look at the cup as being half full, not half empty. Positive vibes are contagious. Enjoy eating well and being active. Feel good about yourself. Have fun with family and friends, and you'll feel on top of the world!"[1]

It's important that children make the connection between health and pleasure. We can help by emphasizing the positive, enjoyable aspects of a healthy lifestyle, and de-emphasizing weight.

Children and teens come in all shapes and sizes. Some store body fat more easily than others. And that's okay. Some stay lean. All bodies are good bodies, whether large or small. Each youngster is special, and we need to accept, respect and celebrate our differences and the ways others differ from us. Some large kids may not be able to change their size, shape or weight much, even though they eat well and live actively. Some will grow into their weight.

We can help kids appreciate their strengths, abilities and unique traits, no matter what their weight. We can help them take pride in themselves and their accomplishments, appreciate the strength and ability of their bodies. We can teach them to appreciate diversity and equality, and to recognize that healthy bodies come in many sizes and shapes. We can help them find useful roles so they feel needed and important at home and in the community. We can also teach young people new ways to relax, to enjoy life and to cope with stress.

When kids feel good about themselves they'll be more likely to feel positive about making healthy changes in their lives.

Eating well

Vitality tells us, "Eating well doesn't mean giving up the foods you love; it means choosing wisely from a variety of foods that you enjoy. Your overall pattern of eating can include foods high, moderate and low in fat. If you want to enjoy a higher-fat food, balance it with staying active and enjoying a wide variety of foods the rest of the day. Children acquire attitudes about food first and foremost at home. Positive attitudes develop when food preparation and mealtimes are pleasant and fun experiences. So take time to enjoy meals and snacks with your children."

When families eat normally — usually three meals with snacks to satisfy hunger — their children are less likely to develop dysfunctional eating patterns. Dieting and restricting moms and dads may have forgotten they can eat moderately, to satisfy hunger and appetite, and yet not eat past the point of satiety.

On the other hand, some kids and their families regularly do eat past the point of satiety or make high-fat food choices. They eat too much food and too much fat, which can cause excess weight gain.

Sometimes we all need to remind ourselves and our children that we feel better if we stop eating when satisfied. The key is to eat enough food to nourish and satisfy, but avoid overeating. At the same time, we can trust our bodies to balance out an occasional episode of overeating, such as a big holiday meal, over a period of days.

All this is part of normal eating.

Enjoying good food

Good foods nourish the body and spirit.

Eating well means choosing from a variety of foods. It means eating that emphasizes choosing fruits and vegetables, whole grains, leaner meats, and lower fat dairy products.

Healthy food choices help youth grow, develop, do well in school, and feel at their best. Even young children can help in buying and preparing food, a practice that helps them make healthy choices at school, with friends, on trips, and later as adults.

Variety, moderation and balance are the guiding principles.

The Food Guide Pyramid helps us visualize the five food groups of bread and grains, fruits, vegetables, the meat group, and milk products.

Eating a variety of foods from all five food groups ensures us of getting the 50-plus essential nutrients for growth, energy and health. A balanced diet, which may be balanced over several days, provides adequate nutrition from each of the five groups. Eating moderately avoids the extremes, eating too much or too little. It reminds us not to overeat on high-fat or high-sugar foods, nor to reject them entirely when they may be favorites. Kids who enjoy a variety of satisfying foods and don't eliminate what they really want are more likely to avoid feelings of deprivation leading to eating problems.

Nutrient-dense foods should be those selected most often from each of the five groups. These are foods high in nutrients and low in calories, fat and added sugars. Many are bulky, high in fiber, and filling — like apples, corn and beans. Others, like eggs, fish or lowfat meats, pack a lot of nutrition into small size and are very satisfying.

Foods that are calorie-dense, not nutrient-dense or bulky — from

Food Guide Pyramid
A Guide to Daily Food Choices

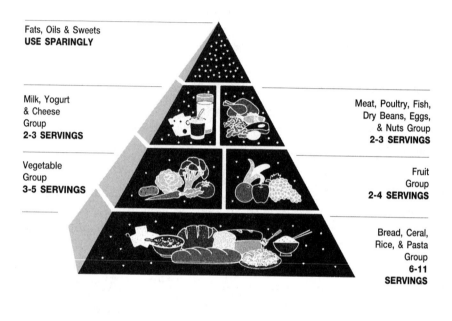

Fats, Oils & Sweets
USE SPARINGLY

Milk, Yogurt
& Cheese
Group
2-3 SERVINGS

Meat, Poultry, Fish,
Dry Beans, Eggs,
& Nuts Group
2-3 SERVINGS

Vegetable
Group
3-5 SERVINGS

Fruit
Group
2-4 SERVINGS

Bread, Ceral,
Rice, & Pasta
Group
**6-11
SERVINGS**

Use the Food Guide Pyramid to help you eat better every day. Start at the pyramid base with plenty of grains, breads, cereals, rice and pasta. At the second level add vegetables and fruits — 5-a-day. Moving up, add two to three servings of milk (three to five for older children and teens) and two to three servings from the meat group. Go easy on or avoid the extra fats, oils and sweets at the tip of the Pyramid, foods which provide calories but few other nutrients.

Eating well focuses on balance, moderation and variety. Balanced food choices come from all five food groups. Eating moderately means eating enough for good nourishment, but not past the point of satiety, and choosing foods that balance out as moderately low in fat and sugars. Eating in variety from each food group ensures you'll get the many nutrients you need for health, energy and growth.[1]

What counts as one serving?
Food Guide Pyramid

Grain products group
- 1 slice of bread
- 1 ounce of ready-to-eat cereal
- 1/2 cup of cooked cereal, rice, or pasta

Vegetable group
- 1 cup of raw leafy vegetables
- 1/2 cup of cooked or chopped raw vegetables
- 3/4 cup vegetable juice

Fruit group
- 1 medium apple, banana, orange
- 1/2 cup of chopped, cooked or canned fruit
- 3/4 cup of fruit juice

Milk group
- 1 cup of milk or yogurt
- 1 1/2 ounces of natural cheese
- 2 ounces of processed cheese

Meat group (meat, poultry, fish, eggs, dry beans, nuts)
- 2-3 ounces of cooked lean meat, poultry or fish
  Equal to 1 ounce of meat, poultry, fish:
    - 1/2 cup cooked dry beans
    - 1 egg
    - 2 tablespoons peanut butter (high in fat)
    - 1/3 cup nuts (high in fat)

In using the pyramid, remember that serving sizes are a general guide. Small children will eat smaller servings; children in a growth spurt, larger teens and older boys may require more and larger servings. Even individuals of the same size differ in the amounts of food they choose and which satisfy their needs. Children should be encouraged to trust their bodies and respond to their natural signals of hunger, appetite and satiety.

DIETARY GUIDELINES FOR AMERICANS/AFRAID TO EAT 1997

the tip of the pyramid — are better eaten less often and in smaller quantity.

The 1995 Dietary Guidelines for Americans offer this advice for healthful eating:

- Eat a variety of foods
- Balance the food you eat with physical activity — maintain or improve your weight
- Choose a diet with plenty of grain products, vegetables and fruits
- Choose a diet low in fat, saturated fat, and cholesterol
- Choose a diet moderate in sugars
- Choose a diet moderate in salt and sodium
- If you drink alcoholic beverages, do so in moderation

It's sound advice for today's youngsters, who rely heavily on processed snack foods, crackers, desserts, candy and soft drinks. They lack adequate fruits and vegetables, and they drink only half the milk and eat less meat and eggs than kids did 15 or 20 years ago.

Improving deficiencies

Surveys suggest that American teens need to improve their diets. Most fail to eat the five-a-day fruits and vegetables recommended. The typical girl or boy over age 11 needs to be drinking much more milk — three to five servings a day from the milk, yogurt and cheese group. (The RDA calls for three servings, but the American Academy of Pediatrics recently raised their recommendation to five for adolescents, to ensure strong bones.) Calcium is essential for healthy bones throughout life and is especially important during the critical bone-building teenage years. If girls don't drink enough milk, and are thin, or often dieting and losing bone mass, they may never develop the strong bones needed to protect them from bone deterioration later in life.

Children who have stopped eating animal source foods like meat, poultry, fish, eggs and milk can benefit greatly from restoring at least some of these to their diets. However, concerned parents need to keep in mind the basic principle that children are responsible for deciding what and how much they will eat. Parents need to respect these decisions, while guiding children toward healthy choices by having a variety of good-tasting foods available. A science-based vegetarian cookbook by credible authors can be helpful.

When parents choose vegetarian diets for themselves and their children, it's important to remember that the more restrictive vegan diets are not recommended for children. It is possible to plan a diet entirely of plant foods that supplies nutrient needs (except for calcium, vitamin B_{12} and vitamin D) but such a diet is so bulky that experts say it is unlikely a young child would eat enough food to get the calories they need, so normal growth may not occur.[2]

Eating at least small amounts of meat has many benefits. Currently there is no basis for suggesting, as some do, that lowering lean meat consumption is healthy, certainly not for children, and it can result in severe deficiencies. The Bogalusa Heart studies found that children who eat more meat are less likely to have nutrient deficiencies than children who eat little or no meat.

In recent years, some writers have claimed the low-meat Mediterranean diet is "ideal" because of longevity in Italy and Greece. But others soon pointed out that people in Sweden and Switzerland live even longer, while consuming diets high in meat and dairy foods.

Eating disorder specialists and pediatricians are seeing alarming numbers of young children with stunted growth, fragile bones and stress fractures who have stopped eating animal products. Some teenage girls have stopped eating meat for fear it may be fattening, but there is no basis for this fear if they choose lean meat and poultry. Research suggests that protein, even in excess, is not stored as fat. And studies show that meals with meat satisfy longer. A Swedish study finds people who eat a meat casserole at lunch, eat fewer calories later in the day than when they eat a vegetable casserole.

Robert Olson, MD, PhD, professor of pediatrics at the University of South Florida, says, "The recommendation to modify the diets of children is without merit."[3]

A diet too low in fat may actually be risky. Fat is not a four-letter word. It's an important nutrient that helps cells use vitamins and minerals more effectively.

It may also be protective. One of the most potent natural

anticarcinogens ever identified in animal studies is conjugated linolic acid, found almost exclusively in animal products, especially milk fat. Cutting out animal fats or animal products will deprive children of whatever cancer preventive benefits they may otherwise get from conjugated linolic acid.[4]

The Dietary Guidelines advise reducing fat intake to 30 percent or less of total calories. This can be easily done if we bring less fat into the house, add less fat in cooking, and use less fat at the table. Cutting down gradually usually works best. For example, spreading half as much table fat on the toast for a few months, later cutting that in half, and perhaps half again, can help us change taste preferences without feeling deprived.

Many kids still have very high fat levels. However, surveys show most have cut down on the fat they eat.

"Good" foods, "bad" foods

When learning to make food choices, kids should be taught that there are no good foods or bad foods. All foods can fit into a healthy eating plan.

The idea that some foods are healthy and others unhealthy suggests that some foods can be used like medicine and others produce disease. This is false and unscientific, although this notion is often promoted in the press, even by health professionals who fail to understand nutrition.

People often use the term "junk foods" to refer to snack foods. But it is well to remember that there are no "junk foods," only "junk diets" — diets that include an over balance of foods from the tip of the pyramid.

While a balanced diet will usually be moderately low in fat and sugars, there's nothing wrong with occasionally eating high-fat, high-sugar foods in the context of an overall healthy food plan. It is important to keep them in balance, or children may fill up on calorie-dense foods and not get needed nutrients.

It's all about you

In making a shift toward health enhancing lifestyles it's helpful to move gradually into new patterns. A national group that advocates this through the new approach of enjoying food, taste and physical activity is the Dietary Guidelines Alliance, a coalition of health organizations, government agencies and food producer groups. The Alliance campaign uses the theme "It's all about you."

The key messages are:

- **Be realistic:** Make small changes over time in what you eat and the level of activity you do. After all, small steps work better than giant leaps.
- **Be adventurous:** Expand your tastes to enjoy a variety of foods.
- **Be flexible:** Go ahead and balance what you eat and the physical activity you do over several days. No need to worry about just one day or one meal.
- **Be sensible:** Enjoy all food, just don't overdo it.
- **Be active:** Walk the dog, don't just watch the dog walk.[5]

How parents can help

In their Iowa extension brochure *A Parent's Guide to Children's Weight,* Carol Hans and Diane Nelson warn that children grow at different rates and may have very different body structures from their own brothers and sisters.[6]

They offer these suggestions on how parents can help children make healthy food choices:

1. Be enthusiastic about eating a variety of foods. Help children learn what foods are in the different food groups and why it's important to eat some of each group daily.
2. Introduce new foods gradually. Offer the child a small portion but do not force the child to eat it. Tasting will come more readily as the food becomes more familiar.
3. Serve realistic portions. The appropriate serving size depends on the child's age and size. One possible guideline is to offer one tablespoon of meat, fruit and vegetable per year of age up to age five. Physical activity and growth spurts also influence appetite. Plan meals to include some lower calorie food items that can be offered for second helpings.
4. Buy fewer high-calorie, low-nutrient foods. Encourage chil-

dren to think of such foods as occasional treats, not regular fare. Involve children in planning, shopping, and label-reading.

Living actively

Active living is widely accepted as a new, broader way of thinking about fitness. Active living is concerned with quality of life and total well-being, not focused on body size.

The Vitality program explains, "Being active means enjoying physical activity and finding fun ways to be active every day of the year — at home, at work, within your community. Whether it's bowling, mowing the lawn or playing hopscotch with the kids, an active lifestyle pays off. Make fitness a family activity: go ice-skating at the local rink, take an after-dinner walk together. Plan an active living vacation — a weekend hike, cross-country ski holiday, a canoeing getaway."

Young children are the most active and physically fit of all Americans. They average one to two hours a day in moderate and vigorous physical activity. And they're active because they want to be, not because it's good for them. Unless we can bring about cultural changes, most will never be this active again. As children grow older, their activity falls off sharply, especially for girls after puberty.

We need to strengthen and extend the joy of activity young children know, and help them carry it into adulthood. It helps to emphasize the pleasure in being active, either alone or with friends. After all, it's just for fun that 12-year-olds play softball all afternoon in a vacant lot. It's for the joy and exhilaration of it that skiers and hikers challenge a mountain. It's for the social and rhythmic, musical pleasure that young people dance nonstop for four hours on a Saturday night.

In this new approach, everyone can succeed, explains Gail Johnston, a health and fitness consultant in Walnut Creek, Calif. It's not necessary to count target heart rates, or calories burned, or work up to training levels. Nor is it necessary to lose weight to achieve the benefits of exercise.[7]

In fact, focusing on weight loss can backfire and take the pleasure out of activity.

So can focusing too much on winning and excelling.

Parents will want to keep tabs on their kids, the teams they play with and coaches they play under, to make sure they're having fun. It's important to create a sense of moderation in sports and active recreation. This keeps the activity fresh, fun and in perspective. It keeps enthusiasm high. Sometimes it's important to cut back on sports or change activities to avoid stress or burnout.

Benefits of exercise

"There are two main reasons why kids should exercise or pursue more physical activities: To be healthy as kids and to increase the probability they will remain physically active as adults," says James Sallis of SPARK.[8]

Being physically active improves health in all sorts of ways. It lowers blood pressure, increases the "good" HDL cholesterol and increases bone density. It lowers stress and anxiety. Regular exercise lifts the mood, and is especially beneficial for youngsters who are depressed or anxious. It relieves tension and helps put problems in perspective.

The effect of exercise on bone density is particularly important during adolescence, because this is the time in life when bone mass peaks.

"Think of the bones as muscles," Sallis suggests. "If you actively use or stress them, the bones will grow stronger."

For example, studies of tennis players show that the arm used most often, the "tennis" arm, has much thicker and stronger bones than the non-tennis arm.

Being active may even make kids smarter. New brain research suggests that exercising the large muscles during adolescence helps increase nerve connections for higher brain development. This supports studies that show students involved in sports do better in academics. They are also less likely to drop out of school, take drugs or get pregnant while in school.

Sports enhance self respect

A recent study by Melpomene Institute and *Shape* magazine of

Healthy People 2000

The Healthy People 2000 midcourse revisions call for increasing the percent of kids of all ages who take daily physical education classes in school. They urge that more time during these classes be spent actively, and that lifetime physical activities be emphasized rather than competitive group sports. Lifetime activities are defined as those that may be readily carried into adulthood and generally need only one or two people, such as swimming, bicycling, jogging, dancing and racquet sports. The Healthy People 2000 objectives as related to youth are as follows:

● Increase the number of children in grades 1-12 who are in daily physical education classes to 75 percent *(from 36 percent in 1984-86).*

● Increase to at least 50 percent the amount of time in school physical education class that students are physically active, preferably in lifetime activities *(from 27 percent in 1983).*

● Increase to at least 30 percent the proportion of people aged 6 and older who engage regularly, preferably daily, in light to moderate physical activity for at least 30 minutes per day.

● Increase to at least 75 percent the proportion of children and adolescents aged 6 through 17 who engage in vigorous physical activity that promotes the development and maintenance of cardiorespiratory fitness 3 or more days per week for 20 or more minutes per occasion. *(Baseline: 66 percent of youth aged 10 through 17 in 1984. For adults increase from 12 percent to 20.)*

● Increase to at least 40 percent the proportion of people aged 6 and older who regularly perform physical activities that enhance and maintain muscular strength, muscular endurance, and flexibility. *(Baseline unavailable)*

● Reduce to no more than 15 percent the proportion of people aged 6 and older who engage in no leisure-time physical activity. *(Especially targeted are blacks, Hispanics, American Indians/Alaska Natives, lower-income people, and people with disabilities.)*

Light to moderate physical activity requires sustained, rhythmic muscular movements, at least equal to sustained walking, performed at less than 60 percent of maximum heart rate for age. Examples are walking, swimming, cycling, dancing, gardening, yardwork, various home activities, games and other childhood pursuits. Vigorous physical activities are rhythmic, repetitive physical activities that use large muscle groups at 60 percent or more of maximum heart rate for age. Maximum heart rate equals roughly 220 beats per minute minus age.[2]

Activity recommendations

People of all ages are advised to engage in:
- Moderate physical activity, accumulating 30 minutes during most days.

For those wanting more benefits, add:
- Vigorous activity for 20 minutes three days a week or more.
- Strength and flexibility exercise three days a week.

Guidelines like these can be helpful. However, the *Vitality* program suggests people shift the focus to being active in their own way, enjoying physical activities as part of their daily lifestyle.

AFRAID TO EAT 1997

---

girls age 11 to 17 found physically active girls were more likely to have high body image, positive sense of self-satisfaction, higher perceived competence, and to like most things about themselves.

Being in athletics enhanced their self respect, and this was increased when they combined sports with other after-school activities. The researchers found that in all cases girls who were in several after-school activities including athletics were more likely to have a higher sense of self than girls involved only in nonphysical activities or no activities. Girls in six or more after-school activities that included athletics were the most likely to feel good about themselves.

The authors suggest that after-school activities offer girls a way to define themselves other than in terms of appearance. They allow girls to develop their interests, become committed, and work with a group toward a common goal — all pursuits unrelated to appearance. The interest and encouragement of parents in their activities also had a big impact on self-esteem measures.[9]

Regular activity appears to be extremely important in preventing obesity for both children and adults. Studies show exercise is also critical in reducing weight and maintaining weight loss over the long term. While these benefits don't show up as quickly as weight loss through restrictive dieting, they last longer.

However, kids and their parents and coaches should avoid a weight loss focus in exercising. The intent should not be to burn as many calories as possible so as to lose weight. This can be self-defeating and lead to dropping out of the activity. So can keeping track of all the dials and measures on fitness equipment, which add up to calories burned and supposedly determine how many pounds will be lost.

This is not really the way it works. In addition, people differ widely in the effect exercise has on their weight.

The role of exercise in weight loss has often been exaggerated, bringing much disappointment and discouragement, warns Chester Zelasko, PhD, director of the Human Performance Laboratory at Buffalo State College in Buffalo, N.Y.[10]

Instead of focusing on exercise for losing weight, he says all people should exercise for the right reasons:

"For the health of it! To improve the cardiovascular system; to improve the strength, endurance and flexibility of the muscular system; to effect positive changes on other body systems such as skeletal, digestive and immune systems; for other manifestations of improved health such as lower serum lipids and lower blood pressure."

Less fit

Most physically underdeveloped youth can become fit if they are motivated. Parents help by understanding the importance of exercise in their child's growth, performance and health, and by getting involved in their children's chosen sports and activities. Parents can also help by limiting television, computer games and browsing, and video time.

While participating in school sports is important, it's clear athletics don't automatically carry over into adulthood. Young athletes have just as great a chance of becoming middle-aged couch potatoes as their non-athletic buddies. In fact, a recent study Sallis conducted at San Diego State University showed the only difference in activity between former high school athletes and non-athletes is that the former athletes watch more televised sports.

Encouraging girls

The roadblocks that still keep many girls from being active in sports need to be removed. Making more facilities available for girls and encouraging girls to use them for pleasure and health will help. This focuses attention on ability and fitness, not appearance, as does the emphasis on weight control.

Research shows that for teenage girls who continue in sports, having fun is their primary motivator. Other motivators are gaining approval and respect, making their parents proud, feeling good about doing well, making friends and keeping in shape, according to Melpomene Institute, a Minneapolis-based group dedicated to physical activity for girls and women.[11]

Women's sports are still under-represented in the media, even though this is changing. It is important for girls to have many good female athlete role models, and to see healthy female athletes of all sizes, not just unnaturally thin women.

It will also help if journalists report on women athletes by emphasizing their ability, strength and skill, instead of exploiting their femininity or appearance.

Exercise programs

In planning an individualized exercise program, Zelasko offers these recommendations for parents and health professionals:

● Emphasize consistency first. Since the goal is to maintain a lifetime of increased physical activity, it is most important to develop the exercise habit. Therefore, before recommending any in-depth, progressive fitness program, develop an easy, minimal workout and ask the person to develop a consistent pattern of activity.

● Encourage duration, intensity and frequency. Consistency is most important, but these factors are also important in building fitness and improving health as the program progresses.

● Intermittent exercise is okay. If the person cannot sustain 10 or 20 minutes at one level, it is okay to break the sessions into segments of alternating low or moderate intensity work — this is interval training, often used by athletes.

● Be a good example. Parents who want their children to gain the benefits of lifetime physical activity are most helpful by modelling what lifetime activity means.

● Respect the large youngster. Everyone deserves respect no matter what his or her body weight. Nurturing is important. Maybe the child will lose weight or grow into the weight. Maybe not. But they can be healthier by exercising regularly and should be reassured of these benefits.

● Understand physical and emotional needs. For kids who have been inactive it takes time to gain confidence in moving the body. They may need to overcome shyness over using their body. As they become more successful, they enjoy activity more, and are more likely to continue. When choosing a fitness facility, it is important to find one where trainers respect the emotional and physical needs of the child.

Parents may want to become involved with their youngsters in helping develop opportunities for community sports activities, safe biking and hiking trails, swimming pools, basketball and tennis courts, and local events and games.

CHAPTER 13

Changing to a
child-friendly culture

■

In a culture that attacks people for being different sizes, we must accept some of the responsibility for allowing the messages. And we must make changes.

If we want our children to grow up in families that love and talk to each other, we can work to provide them. If we want our children to grow up with solid, positive self respect and body images, we can work to encourage them. If we want girls to grow up free from sexual harassment, then we can stop it.

If we want the media to reflect to us images of healthy people in a variety of sizes, then we can work toward that. If we want our children, who are afraid to eat or who overeat, to grow up eating normally and making healthy lifestyle choices, then we can support these choices.

Families, communities and schools

Changing culture is a huge task, but it's possible. Strong forces have molded today's society, and change won't be easy, nor will it happen overnight.

Changing our society into one that values healthy living, women, and many body sizes, means enlisting families, schools and communities.

There are signs people are ready for a change.

The mood of the nation is swinging toward a yearning for stronger "family values," and safer and more nurturing communities. Politicians in both major parties are taking up the cause of strengthening the family and lessening the impact of destructive elements.

Worldwide, there is backlash against fashion's severe excesses in portraying malnutrition as glamorous, although the industry's resistance to change is strong.

When the Omega watch company decided to pull its ads from the British *Vogue* in protest against two extremely thin models, the public and media overwhelmingly supported the Swiss watchmaker. The magazine featured "skeletal" waifs Annie Morton and Trish Goff modeling underwear and sportswear in body-revealing poses.

Giles Rees, British Omega marketing manager, said the photos would encourage eating disorders in young women. "It was irresponsible for a leading magazine, which should be setting an example, to select models of anorexic proportions."

However, Omega's chairman, Nicolas Hayek, overruled Rees and reinstated the advertising. British *Vogue* arrogantly lauded the decision as a triumph.

"A complete victory!" crowed *Vogue* publisher Stephen Quinn. "It's good news in terms of editorial independence."

I hope Giles Rees will speak out again as strongly, and that he and others will follow their consciences in advertising. The more support they get from us, the public, the more likely they will do this.

Female diversity in role models

It's important to be presenting healthier images of girls and women in the media and public life, as real people with diverse talents, of varied sizes, ages and shapes, deserving of respect regardless of whether they are glamorous or not. Girls need these role models.

Today's beauty standards are so narrow that women in the media all seem to look alike — hollow-cheeked, passive, focused on their appearance, vulnerable and extremely thin. They appear as decorative or sexual objects to be admired, used or discarded. It's a stereotype that sets 9-year-olds dieting and teaches adolescent girls that their developing bodies will never be good enough. It compels young girls to live as if they are being constantly watched, desired, judged.

As women move into decision-making positions in the media, I have hoped this situation would improve of itself. Unfortunately, despite the many advances made by women, this has not happened. Women's stereotyping in the media shows no signs of improving.

It is time that women who are producers, editors, reporters, models and actresses make this needed shift. Girls and women are not objects or toys, and it is most unfortunate when preteen and teen girls are led to believe this is their role. Young people need to be liberated from these false and narrow images based on appearances.

I've been encouraged by the publicity given the outstanding 1996 Olympic women's athletic teams in softball, basketball and track events. I was encouraged (and astounded) by the 1997 Academy Awards selection of Frances McDormand as best actress of the year in the movie *Fargo,* looking much like America's ordinary women, getting up early, going about her day's work, albeit unique work, in big furry bomber hat, ear lappers flopping, with nary a seductive smile. It has to be a first ever for the Academy! I appreciate entertainers like Rosie O'Donnell, Oprah Winfrey and Roseanne. I also applaud public figures like Attorney General Janet Reno who, when she appears on television, doesn't look as if she's spent the last four hours in the beauty shop, but rather working in her office, like women everywhere.

Do these examples signal more of a willingness to reveal the diversity of women? Or does their rarity only prove again that major decision-makers just don't get it?

Girl's teen magazines need to change their focus from today's tiresome replay. Stories on makeup, fashion, weight loss and how to attract boys may be topics of enormous interest to their advertisers but are hardly challenging for girls. They need to include more stories on sports, careers, hobbies, and credible young women doing interesting things. Or be replaced by magazines that do, so that girls are no longer led to "sacrifice their true selves" for lookism.

I personally try to encourage a wider portrayal of women's diversity by giving special awards on Women's Healthy Weight Day. Every third Thursday in January, during Healthy Weight Week, we at *Healthy Weight Journal* honor television shows, networks, magazines, advertisers and businesses that portray non-stereotypical women and confirm that beauty, health and strength come in all sizes. Numerous radio talk show hosts feature this event on their shows, and we field questions from reporters and journalists worldwide who are delighted with the concept.

I believe that if a few leading teen and women's magazines will have the courage to depict girls and women of all sizes in their pages, the unhealthy media stereotypes can change rapidly. Other editors, television producers, and Hollywood itself will be stunned to discover the beauty, charm and unique talents of real women in all their diversity — and their popularity with the public.

One beauty magazine that seems to be providing some leadership in this area is *Glamour*. In 1997 we gave *Glamour* a Women's Healthy Weight Day media award for publishing articles on glamorous larger women and initiating a feature for women of all sizes.[1]

A positive influence may be the new freedom of exchange offered by the Internet, in which communication counts most and appearance is irrelevant.

Advertising and the media

Taking on the media — television, movies, books, magazines, newspapers, advertising, billboards, music — will not be easy. But the media carry many destructive messages about body size, sexuality and women that affect all areas of our lives. Multinational companies advertising throughout the world have seized unprecedented power in creating body dissatisfaction and negatively impacting culture everywhere.

Regardless of difficulty, cultural changes can be made. Psychologist Mary Pipher says in *Reviving Ophelia* that we can help girls fight cultural pressures, encourage their emotional toughness and self-protection, and strengthen and guide them.[2]

"Most important, we can change our culture. We can work together to build a culture that is less complicated and more nurturing, less violent and sexualized and more growth-producing. Our daughters deserve a society in which all their gifts can be developed and appreciated."

She warns that it is critically important to change the way women are portrayed in the media, as expensive toys, the ultimate recreation, "half-clad and half-witted, often awaiting rescue by quick-thinking, fully clothed men . . ."

People concerned with these issues can work together to change the focus of responsible media and advertising, and to deflate the poisonous influence of its irresponsible fringe.

The media can be encouraged to portray healthy lifestyles and healthy female images, and supported when they do. I'd like to see a great outpouring of support for positive portrayals and a boycotting of the offensive.

The focus on malnourished bodies for women can be reversed. It is clear from several studies that fashion's ideal female is continuing to grow thinner. The incident at *Vogue* shows these pressures are increasing, not abating, as has been rumored.

Parents and consumer groups can be vigilant in making strong complaints against destructive stereotyping in magazines, television and advertising.

A boycott can be extremely effective.

It worked for a Boston-based consumer group that calls itself "BAM" (Boycott Anorexic Marketing). BAM forced the cancelation of Diet Sprite ads that depicted a bony, apathetic girl sipping a diet drink, boasting her nickname was "Skeleton."

BAM's Diet Sprite boycott was picked up on national news and Coca Cola hastily pulled the Diet Sprite ads.

Letters, phone calls, faxes, e-mail and internet messages are effective in combatting these destructive images. Targeting offensive advertisers is important, and their advertising mediums should not be let off easy, either. When magazines print these ads or stations air them, they are responsible for what they give their audience. Editors keep a wary eye on marketing and routinely slant articles to please their advertisers, often to the detriment of the public, as in the case of smoking. They can be pressured to instead edit for what their readers demand.

On a more impulsive note, vigilantes are striking at offensive displays on billboards and buses by scrawling graffiti over thin women's bodies.

"I'm So Hungry," lamented the caption on one gaunt model.

"Please Give Me a Cheeseburger," another pleaded.

It is true that one person can make a difference, three or four together can make a miracle. A nation motivated to action can bring about an attitude change overnight.

"Never doubt that a handful of committed individuals can truly change the world," said anthropologist Margaret Mead.

It is my hope that readers of this book will be inspired to initiate changes aimed at respecting the diversity of women.

Inoculate with education

Schools can do much to diffuse the power of advertising by training students how to protect their self concepts from narrow media stereotypes, beginning in preadolescence where media images have such powerful impact.

Even young children can understand the advertisers' self-interest in creating body dissatisfaction to sell products. Our children do not have to be pawns in this game. They can learn the pervasive technique of focusing on extremes to make products stand out: "if long legs are good, our models have longer and thinner legs; if wide spaced eyes and hollow cheeks are good, ours are spaced wider, our cheeks more gaunt than have ever been seen before."

They can determine for themselves that these extreme images do not provide healthy role models for real youngsters who have real lives and interesting futures. They will respond to clear messages that this exploitation is not acceptable to adults or peers.

Demonstrating the ease with which photos are computerized today should make these images less attractive and less believable as role models. Consumer education for youngsters at all levels can include hands-on projects on how to evaluate television and print advertising. Training workshops for leaders can also be helpful.

Girls, in particular, can learn to be skeptical of advertising, the dieting culture, and the language of advertising which suggests that a woman's body and face always needs fixing — it's never quite good enough.

Girls can also be helped to recognize how media images constrain not just their body shape, but their behavior.

Gail Huon, a psychologist at the University of South Wales in Sydney, Australia, writes in the journal *Eating Disorders* that girls must be taught to critically review the media images, articles and advertising not only for female thinness, but also for passiveness and submissiveness. They need to examine how women are portrayed in advertising as "property," and as waiting, receptive, ready to contribute to someone else's life.

In doing this, they can reclaim their lives and see their real choices and options. Young women can be helped to respond positively to the challenges of their environment in order to achieve their potential, she says.[3]

Protecting youth from abuse

Eating disorders and other disturbed and dysfunctional eating patterns may begin as ways of coping with the trauma, violence, sexual abuse, physical abuse, harassment, bullying or stigmatization that is pervasive in our culture, and even glamorized in the media. Working together, communities, schools and families can protect our young people from these violations of the self, which can impact eating and weight in harmful ways.

Youth who are singled out for special torment by their peers, or stigmatized because of their size, appearance, disability, homosexuality, or ethnicity deserve protection by the adults in their lives.

The National Education Association has declared itself ready to combat size prejudice in the schools. The largest teacher organization in the country launched its investigation of size discrimination in schools as a human and civil rights issue in 1993. The ensuing NEA report described the school experience as one of "ongoing prejudice, unnoticed discrimination, and almost constant harassment" for large students.

"This situation can be changed by education employees who are sensitive to America's obsession with the thin and intolerance toward the fat. They can foster a better learning and growing environment for students with unique needs due to size."

In 1994 NEA pledged to "continue to support efforts to foster an improved teaching and learning environment for colleagues and students who have special needs due to physical size; further, that NEA review its existing policies and recommend policy revisions in this regard, as appropriate."[4]

I hope teachers and school personnel will soon move this policy forward in their local schools. Although most of the NEA members I talk with are unfamiliar with the report, they seem eager to support a policy of zero tolerance for size bias in schools.

Sexual harassment

Sexual harassment is one of the important ways in which young girls' pleasure about their developing bodies is destroyed, experts say. It can alienate them from self, cause them to "hate" their bodies as a separate part of themselves, and oppress them with an overwhelming sense of shame.

Sexual harassment is seldom discussed, so victims bear their shame in secret. Boys, showing off for their peers, may not understand the harm they inflict with "clever" remarks. Girls, too, may be the harrassers in many cases.

For both girls and boys, consciousness-raising groups can be enlightening and empowering. Girls are often surprised to find they have had common harassing experiences with other girls that have little to do with what they fear are their personal inadequacies.

In Toronto, Carla Rice and Vanessa Russell, Women's Studies specialists at the Ontario Institute for Studies in Education, organized support groups for girls on body image and body equity. They were asked to document gender oppression in the public schools, and to develop equity and health education programs for the Toronto Board of Education.[5]

In their early focus groups, they report, no one wanted to talk. Then one young woman would cautiously tell an incident she thought might be sexual harassment. Others declared the same thing had happened to them, "and then the stories flowed."

The girls felt relief when they found the courage to talk and realized they were not alone. Then they grew outraged as they connected the shame they felt about their bodies to incidents of violence or harassment. Each had endured her humiliation in secret, ashamed to tell anyone, because she feared she either deserved or had provoked the hurtful comments.

Rice and Russell watched the girls' shame turn to anger and their self-loathing to acceptance as they realized most other girls had the same experiences with harassment. This shift from shame to anger may be a key to empowerment, they suggest. It's a transition from "I deserve to be violated," to "I have been violated," to "I do not deserve and will not tolerate violation."

As they shared their experiences, the girls grew more affirming and appreciative of each other, and became "a force to be reckoned with."

Can you imagine girls and their parents and teachers being a force to be reckoned with across the country in not allowing size bias or sexual harassment? I can, and it would make a big difference.

Consider this scenario: A group of girls (or both girls and boys) decides to stick together and take action. Instead of silently and individually absorbing the abuse when other students make disparaging remarks in the school hallway, they consider it an opportunity to document what's going on. They take out their notebooks and write it all down — date, time, who said what, or did what. With this documentation over a period of several weeks, they present their case to school officials, teachers, counselors, parents, clergy and other adults willing to listen. Following through with effective action proves to themselves that they are not powerless, and just getting together to talk about what's happening can help to dispel the shame they feel.

As a result of their work, Rice and Russell encourage wider discussion of these issues among those who work with teenagers. They urge group programs to provide girls with tools to fight against the weapons of oppression, including giving them alternative images that celebrate women's diversity, providing and sharing stories of resistance and empowerment, and instilling a sense of pride in their bodies and themselves.

Boys as well as girls can be taught to recognize sexual harassment and know its consequences. They need to know what is not acceptable — so boys don't go on to become the men whose firms are sued for sexual harassment and they can't understand why.

Educating both boys and girls in how to be loving and gentle can help curb violence and harassment.

It has been said that there are no rules in sexual behavior — until they are broken. This is true for young men as well as young women. When rules are broken, it's as if the offenders should have known all along what is acceptable, and they may feel betrayed because they didn't know.

Young people also need to know that perpetrators will be held responsible for their actions. Potential abusers need to clearly understand the impact of what they do. They need to be taught ways to control their behavior and develop more appropriate ways of communicating or coping.

This type of education may not fit easily into a society such as ours which flaunts sexuality and the availability of sex, but has many taboos and fears of talking about sexuality and abusive sexual incidents. Yet it is imperative that ways be found to do this. Local decisions made with parents seems the best way to deal with such subjects.

Prevention efforts will also address the cultural structures that promote sexual exploitation and the manipulation of children's and women's bodies.

For example, why do we still dote on beauty contests for little girls and teens, putting their young bodies on display, even bared for swimsuit competitions? Charles Dinn, publisher of *Pageantry* magazine, estimates that 100,000 children under the age of 12 perform in U.S. beauty pageants every year. There must be other venues for showcasing the talents of these girls. And how can we allow these pageants to dictate, as they allegedly attempted to do with the 1996 Miss Universe, that a girl is too fat if she's 5-foot-7 and weighs 130 pounds?

Preventing sexual abuse

It is the responsibility of adults — parents, teachers and institutional personnel, as well as potential perpetrators — to protect children from sexual abuses. This places the moral, ethical and legal responsibility where it belongs, with the adults surrounding the child.

Parents, teachers, volunteers and administrative and other staff can all be educated in the detection, handling and reporting of child sexual abuse. When crimes are committed, it is the responsibility of law enforcement to separate the criminal from potential victims and to inform communities of convicted offenders in their midst. Our children must be protected from sexually aggressive predators.

Kids can be taught effective and safe ways of defending themselves against sexual aggressors, whether of the same age, older youth, or adults. But this does not imply that children are responsible for preventing their own abuse.

Experts advise airing public service messages like these:

■ Sexual molestation of children is a crime.

■ A child is unable to give consent.

■ Sexual molestation of children involves an abuse of power and trust that is based on coercion and intimidation.

■ Sexual molestation is damaging to children.

■ Preventing sexual abuse is the exclusive responsibility of adults.

As adults we need to stop sexual abusers and hold them accountable for their crimes. Treatment programs can help offenders understand the impact of their abusive behavior and learn more appropriate alternative behaviors. Drugs or surgery may be considered as well as behavior therapy in treatment programs.

Abuse may occur where it is least expected. Stermac, Piran and Sheridan warn of incest. They recommend that first-time parents be targeted for intervention, informed about appropriate and inappropriate touching, and how to detect in oneself and one's mate the inclination toward inappropriate touching and what to do about it. They advise informing parents of the high incidence of sexual abuse within the family or by close relatives, the tendency to deny abuse, and how to build a protective environment for their children. Discussing healthy sexuality with children may provide opportunities to identify abnormal and destructive sexual situations within a positive context.

"Young men need to be socialized in such a way that rape is as unthinkable to them as cannibalism," writes Pipher.

She points out that rape hurts everyone, not just its victims. It keeps all women in a state of fear about men. Men are fearful for their women friends and aware that women are afraid of them. But mostly rape damages young women. Pipher quotes statistics that show 41 percent of rape victims expect to be raped again; 30 percent contemplate suicide; 31 percent go into therapy, and 82 percent say their lives are permanently changed.

Pipher says the incidence of rape is increasing because of our culture's increasingly destructive messages about sexuality. "Sex is currently associated with violence, power, domination and status."

What needs to happen, I think, is for women to break their silence, reveal their stories, stop protecting the men who have abused them, and tell their young daughters (and sons) you don't have to put up with sexual abuse, if it happens we'll deal with it together, I'll believe you, I'll help you.

This may be a way to free victims from the sense of shame and powerlessness. Can it happen? Why not? We've come an amazing distance since the mid-1980s, when incest or even sexual harassment was hardly spoken aloud.

Stop fearmongering

Reducing media confusion and fearmongering over health and food issues would help children and their families eat normally again.

Elizabeth Whelan, president of the American Council on Science and Health calls on scientists, policy makers, the media and consumers to stop the fearmongering and implement changes such as the following:[6]

■ Emphasize that our food supply is safe. Keep reassuring the press and public of the truth: that America has the safest, healthiest, most enviable food supply in the world. The rarity of adverse incidents should be used to prove, rather than dispute, this fact.

■ Return to mainstream science that defends reason and rationality. Whelan says many scientists don't want to get involved, and yet they must. And they must communicate, not in uncertainties as scientists are wont to do, but in easily understandable terms that make clear what the relative risks are.

■ Emphasize healthy nutrition messages and insist on balance. Restore acceptance of the basic principle that health depends on the total diet, not on a few special components. Convey the message that all foods can fit into a healthy diet. All the five food groups in variety are important for healthy, balanced nutrition. Further, there are no "bad" foods. Even high-fat foods, the current bugaboo, can be balanced by low-fat foods.

■ Diffuse the power to grab headlines of "health terrorists" and "food terrorists," whether these are ill-informed consumer groups, journalists on a "politically correct" mission, talk show hosts seeking higher ratings, radical animal rights groups, or scientists shoring up their grant funding. Whelan calls them spokesmen from the "Chicken Little School of Environmental Hyperbole." They need to be exposed as such.

■ Expose the corruption of "politically correct science." This trendy ideology makes environmentalism and consumerism the new religion, says Whelan. It is against industry, technology, and free enterprise. It abandons science, reason and rationality. It is an ideology which has infused the press with false notions that American health is at risk from additives, preservatives and substances used to increase food production. There is no scientific evidence to suggest that any of these are health risks.

■ Reduce the influence of the tobacco industry to silence criticism and divert attention from the real health risks. When over 1,300 Americans die prematurely every day from tobacco, and some 300 die of the affects of alcohol every day, it is almost ludicrous that nonrisks get the major headlines. Tobacco has privileged status which needs to be stripped. It is time to stop the power of smoking advertisements and acknowledge that the billions of dollars spent on advertising have been effective in silencing most smoking criticism in magazines and newspapers.

As consumers we can just tune out these "health terrorist" headlines and encourage kids to do the same, knowing that most headline stories are jumping on sensational, improbable or unknown risks.

CHAPTER 14

Call to action

■

It's time to develop a vision and direction. This is an urgent challenge for America and countries around the world.

We need to deal with the current weight and eating crisis in healthy ways — ways that don't repeat the mistakes of the past.

The unified health approach recognizes the interrelatedness of four major problems: dysfunctional eating, eating disorders, overweight and size prejudice. It furthers healthy growth and development of the whole child in mind, body and spirit, and it includes every child of every size.

The process of developing this unified vision needs to involve parents, teachers, health care providers, policy makers and specialists, people of insight, intelligence, integrity, and an understanding of the special concerns of women and minorities.[1]

How can we reach a shared vision and effectively communicate that vision? How can we promote wellness and wholeness in positive ways for children of all sizes?

Challenges for wellness and wholeness

The unified health approach challenges us to make changes in these five areas: attitude, lifestyle, prevention, health care, and knowledge.

1. Attitude

The new approach advocates a shift in attitudes toward:

■ Wider awareness and concern for weight and eating issues, for their interrelatedness, and their importance in children's healthy growth and development.

■ Greater appreciation for healthy lifestyles and balanced, wholesome living (versus being thin) to help people feel encouraged to make healthy changes in their own lives. Appreciating the pleasurable, energizing and healthful benefits.

■ Less concern for appearance, and more for respect, character, responsibility, achievement, family and community. Conveying to girls and women who may be fixated on appearance that when well nourished they can live richer, more interesting lives.

■ Intolerance for violations against persons, such as harassment, stigmatization, and mental, physical and sexual abuse.

■ Acceptance of a wider range of sizes, appreciation of diversity, and recognition that beauty comes in all shapes and sizes. Rejecting extreme thinness (or any shape) as the "ideal" body type.

■ Increased determination to deal with negative aspects of the media through education, political action and possible boycotting. Diffusing advertising's focus on body dissatisfaction and appearance as a way to sell products. Insisting the news media report health news more responsibly, putting it into perspective of how much risk there really is (compared to smoking, for example). Exposing health terrorists and unsound "politically correct" views, rather than perpetuating them.

■ Recognition of the media as a powerful instrument for positive attitude change. Enlisting and supporting the media in providing worthy role models. Strong, talented, intelligent women of diverse sizes, ages and ethnicity need to be much more visible in the entertainment industries and public life to provide role models for our daughters and female figures of respect for our sons.

2. Lifestyle

The new approach promotes healthy lifestyles which embrace:

- Pleasurable, normal eating and a moderate, varied, balanced diet, moderately low in fat, avoiding extremes.
- Active living. Improving physical education programs in schools and motivating youth to continue being active through life. Encouraging active living in the U.S. through a national public health program as in many advanced countries.
- Promoting the attainment and maintenance of genetically favorable weights for growing children, and natural, stable weights for adults. Stopping dieting and ineffective, unsafe weight loss practices.
- Managing stress levels. Teaching effective ways to reduce and manage stress. Enhancing self respect, self acceptance, feelings of being needed, and positive relations with family, friends, community. Focusing on balance, moderation and contentment with life. Avoiding extremes.
- Reducing violence, sexual abuse, harassment and stigmatization, particularly against children and young girls. Finding effective ways to protect girls from aggressive men. Providing more counseling accessibility and support for victims. Increasing law enforcement and incarceration to separate abusers from potential victims.
- Promoting environments that support being active, eating well, reducing stress and appreciating size diversity through schools, health care providers, the community, media and home. Communities can do much to encourage active living: developing safe, well-lighted playgrounds, parks, swimming pools, skating rinks, and trails for walking, bicycling and cross-country skiing. They can open school gymnasiums to the public, provide recreation centers, and organize community fitness campaigns and events.

3. Prevention

The health paradigm emphasizes prevention of the four weight and eating problems (dysfunctional eating, eating disorders, overweight and size prejudice) through:

- Promoting healthy attitudes and healthy lifestyles as discussed in the two preceding sections.
- Developing special prevention programs for school and community, being certain that they will do no harm. Recognizing the grave concerns about adopting preventive programs prematurely, without adequate research into safety and effectiveness, these steps are suggested:
  1. Develop goals aimed at three levels: (a) prevention of weight and eating problems for all youngsters, (b) identification of and possible intervention for youth with eating and weight problems in early stages, while avoiding stigmatizing them, (c) referral of individuals with severe problems to specialists.
  2. Develop and pilot test programs, including culture-specific programs for high-risk minority, ethnic, and income groups. Evaluate and report results, including benefits and potentially harmful effects. Determine course of action through networking with other researchers, specialists and local leaders.
  3. Fine-tune and implement programs. Continue to test and evaluate available programs.

4. Health care

A health promoting shift in national policy and local health care services will:

- Ensure that health professionals consistently promote healthy lifestyles and being healthy at every size. Focus on improving the health of large individuals, not on ineffective weight loss. Stop submitting large children to diets, drugs, and weight loss surgery without proof of long-term safety and effectiveness; they have time to wait for safe and effective methods.
- Reduce size prejudice in health care. Many health care providers need to be aware of and work to overcome their own biases, so that large patients can come to them with the assurance of respectful treatment.

■ Identify and treat dysfunctional eating at early stages, not waiting for clinical eating disorder diagnoses.

■ Improve access to qualified services for high-risk populations.

■ Regulate obesity treatment, as other health-related procedures. Require adequate safety and effectiveness studies before going ahead with treatment. Require full disclosure and accountability, reporting weight loss results, adverse effects, morbidity and mortality. See Connecticut law for model regulations.[2]

■ Add eating disorders to the priorities for health promotion and disease prevention for Healthy People 2010, establishing objectives, baselines and measurable targets.

■ Develop a sound policy on use of weight loss drugs, since the potential for abuse now and in the future is high. Require credible studies demonstrating long-term safety and effectiveness, not one-year studies, as today. Begin dialogue on ethical use of drugs: When effective drugs are available will it be ethical to prescribe them widely, for children as well as adults? Should they be available without prescription?[3]

5. Knowledge

The new unified health approach in meeting challenges for research and information will:

■ Encourage dietetics and nutrition schools to develop programs and support groups to deal effectively with the high levels of dysfunctional eating now found among college students, including students in their own departments. Develop more extensive courses in weight and eating issues at undergraduate and graduate levels.

■ Encourage medical schools to require basic studies in nutrition, obesity and eating disorders. At the same time, promote more reliance by doctors on nutritionists and others with special training in these areas, and the referring of patients to specialists.

■ Consolidate eating and weight studies into one academic department within a field such as nutrition or health, developing graduate programs to train specialists. This will move the field ahead more rapidly. Bringing these now-fragmented issues together into a respected field of study will mean the information is researched, analyzed and used in more comprehensive ways. Also, the power of vested interests will be lessened.

■ Communicate research and information in more comprehensive, health-promoting ways to health professionals and consumers.

■ Encourage female researchers in their efforts to report at conferences, publish in scientific literature, and take leadership positions. Domination by patriarchal males in research, publishing, scientific conferences, and health care has prevented this in the past, and delayed recognition of the importance of women's concerns, such as the role of sexual abuse in eating disorders.

■ Raise ethical standards. Require full disclosure of funding and commercial relationships at scientific conferences, on journal editorial boards and in public policy, to reduce the influence of the weight loss industry. (Obesity research has been particularly vulnerable to vested interests, resulting in charges of manipulation of data, evasion of full disclosure, and reporting of short-term, irrelevant findings as if they were lasting and important.) Require truthful reporting, in the public's best interest, and drop the fiction that current obesity treatments are safe and effective.

■ Increase research into the four major problems (dysfunctional eating, eating disorders, overweight, size prejudice), their etiology, causes, treatment and prevention. Learn more about normal eating; body regulation of weight, hunger, appetite and satiety; the physical and mental effects of starvation and semi-starvation; the nature of the "thrifty gene" and how it impacts populations undergoing cultural change.

On a personal note

Each of us has the power to bring about change in our lives. It is my hope that readers of this book will make positive shifts to the new health approach in personal, professional and policy areas, and will consider making personal commitments in two areas. For some this will be easy, or they're already there; for others it may be extremely difficult. I'm confident this shift will be worthwhile and, since each of us is a role model, will help bring about change in others.

The first suggestion is to practice normal eating. This means eating at regular times, usually three meals a day and snacks to satisfy hunger. It means rediscovering hunger, appetite and satiety, and trusting our own instincts. It means developing reasonable habits and getting on with life.

The second suggestion is to promote "zero tolerance for size bias." What will this mean for our attitudes and behavior? How will it affect the way we relate to others, both the victims of prejudice and their oppressors? I'm not suggesting continual confrontation of the bully. But sometimes it may be appropriate to say, "Stop. Everyone deserves respect and you need to respect Jane as a fellow human being." And sometimes Jane needs our words of comfort and support, either at the time or later, in private. She'll feel less alone. And we'll feel better. Size discrimination hurts us all, and especially vulnerable children, because it means no one is ever thin enough to be "safe." Taking a stand against this has a powerful effect.

Working together, we can shift our national focus to the goal of healthy children of all sizes, to wellness and wholeness for the whole child and every child. We can develop a unified health approach in which all children and teens receive consistent messages that encourage normal eating, active living, self respect and an appreciation of size diversity. We can help them grow and develop in ways that enhance their intellectual, emotional, physical, social and spiritual well-being. We can free our children and help them fulfill their potential as generous, capable, unique individuals.

Body Mass Index for Selected Weight and Stature

Stature m (in)

Weight kg (lb)	1.24 (49)	1.27 (50)	1.30 (51)	1.32 (52)	1.35 (53)	1.37 (54)	1.40 (55)	1.42 (56)	1.45 (57)	1.47 (58)	1.50 (59)	1.52 (60)	1.55 (61)	1.57 (62)	1.60 (63)	1.63 (64)	1.65 (65)	1.68 (66)	1.70 (67)	1.73 (68)	1.75 (69)	1.78 (70)	1.80 (71)	1.83 (72)	1.85 (73)	1.88 (74)	1.90 (75)	1.93 (76)
20 (45)	13	13	12	12	11	11	10	10	10	10	9	9	9	8														
23 (50)	15	14	13	13	12	12	12	11	11	10	10	10	9	9	9	9	8											
25 (55)	16	15	15	14	14	13	13	12	12	12	11	11	10	10	10	9	9	9										
27 (60)	18	17	16	16	15	15	14	13	13	13	12	12	11	11	11	10	10	10	9	9								
29 (65)	19	18	17	17	16	16	15	15	14	14	13	13	12	12	12	11	11	10	10	10	10							
32 (70)	21	20	19	18	17	17	16	16	15	15	14	14	13	13	12	12	12	11	11	11	10	10						
34 (75)	22	21	20	20	19	18	17	17	16	16	15	15	14	14	13	13	12	12	12	11	11	11	10					
36 (80)	24	22	21	21	20	19	19	18	17	17	16	16	15	15	14	14	13	13	13	12	12	11	11	11				
39 (85)	25	24	23	22	21	21	20	19	18	18	17	17	16	16	15	15	14	14	13	13	13	12	12	12	11			
41 (90)	27	25	24	23	22	22	21	20	19	19	18	18	17	17	16	15	15	14	14	14	13	13	13	12	12	12		
43 (95)	28	27	25	25	24	23	22	21	20	20	19	19	18	17	17	16	16	15	15	14	14	13	13	13	12	12		
45 (100)	29	28	27	26	25	24	23	22	22	21	20	20	19	18	18	17	17	16	16	15	15	14	14	14	13	13	13	12
48 (105)	31	30	28	27	26	25	24	24	23	22	21	21	20	19	19	18	17	17	16	16	16	15	15	14	14	13	13	13
50 (110)	32	31	30	29	27	27	25	25	24	23	22	22	21	20	19	19	18	18	17	17	16	16	15	15	15	14	14	13
52 (115)	34	32	31	30	29	28	27	26	25	24	23	23	22	21	20	20	19	18	18	17	17	16	16	16	15	15	14	14
54 (120)	35	34	32	31	30	29	28	27	26	25	24	24	23	22	21	20	20	19	19	18	18	17	17	16	16	15	15	15
57 (125)	37	35	34	33	31	30	29	28	27	26	25	24	23	22	21	21	20	20	19	18	18	17	17	17	16	16	16	
59 (130)	38	37	35	34	32	31	30	29	28	27	26	26	25	24	23	22	22	21	20	20	19	19	18	18	17	17	16	16
61 (135)	40	38	36	35	34	33	31	30	29	28	27	27	25	25	24	23	22	22	21	20	20	19	19	18	18	17	17	16
64 (140)	41	39	38	36	35	34	32	31	30	29	28	27	26	26	25	24	23	22	22	21	21	20	20	19	19	18	18	17
66 (145)	43	41	39	38	36	35	34	33	31	30	29	28	27	27	26	25	24	23	23	22	21	21	20	20	19	19	18	18
68 (150)	44	42	40	39	37	36	35	34	32	31	30	29	28	28	27	26	25	24	24	23	22	21	21	20	20	19	19	18
70 (155)	46	44	42	40	39	37	36	35	33	33	31	30	29	29	27	26	26	25	24	23	23	22	22	21	21	20	19	19
73 (160)	47	45	43	42	40	39	37	36	35	34	32	31	30	29	28	27	27	26	25	24	24	23	22	22	21	21	20	19
77 (170)	50	48	46	44	42	41	39	38	37	36	34	33	32	31	30	29	28	27	27	26	25	24	24	23	23	22	21	21
79 (175)		49	47	46	44	42	40	39	38	37	35	34	33	32	31	30	29	28	27	27	26	25	24	24	23	22	22	21
82 (180)		51	48	47	45	44	42	40	39	38	36	35	34	33	32	31	30	29	28	27	27	26	25	24	24	23	23	22
84 (185)			50	48	46	45	43	42	40	39	37	36	35	34	33	32	31	30	29	28	27	26	26	25	25	24	23	23
86 (190)				49	47	46	44	43	41	40	39	37	36	35	34	32	32	31	30	29	28	27	27	26	25	24	24	23
88 (195)				51	49	47	45	44	42	41	39	38	37	36	35	33	33	32	31	30	29	28	27	27	26	25	25	24
91 (200)					50	48	46	45	43	42	40	39	38	37	35	34	33	32	31	30	30	29	28	27	27	26	25	24
93 (205)						50	47	46	44	43	41	40	39	38	36	35	34	33	32	31	30	29	29	28	27	26	26	25
95 (210)							49	47	45	44	42	41	40	39	37	36	35	34	33	32	31	30	29	28	28	27	26	26
98 (215)							50	48	46	45	43	42	41	40	38	37	36	35	34	33	32	31	30	29	28	28	27	26
100 (220)								49	47	46	44	43	42	40	39	38	37	35	35	33	33	31	31	30	29	28	28	27
102 (225)								51	49	47	45	44	42	41	40	38	37	36	35	34	33	32	31	30	30	29	28	27
104 (230)									50	48	46	45	43	42	41	39	38	37	36	35	34	33	32	31	30	30	29	28
107 (235)										49	47	46	44	43	42	40	39	38	37	36	35	34	33	32	31	30	30	29
109 (240)										50	48	47	45	44	43	41	40	39	38	36	36	34	34	33	32	31	30	29
111 (245)											49	48	46	45	43	42	41	39	38	37	36	35	34	33	32	31	31	30
113 (250)											50	49	47	46	44	43	42	40	39	38	37	36	35	34	33	32	31	30
116 (255)												50	48	47	45	44	43	42	40	39	38	37	36	35	34	33	32	31
118 (260)													49	48	46	44	43	42	41	39	39	37	36	35	34	33	33	32
120 (265)													50	49	47	45	44	43	42	40	39	38	37	36	35	34	33	32
122 (270)														50	48	46	45	43	42	41	40	39	38	37	36	35	34	33
125 (275)															49	48	46	44	43	42	41	40	39	38	37	36	35	35
127 (280)															50	48	47	45	44	42	41	40	39	38	37	36	35	34
129 (285)															50	49	47	46	45	43	42	41	40	39	38	37	36	35
132 (290)																50	48	47	46	44	43	42	41	39	38	37	36	35
134 (295)																50	49	47	46	45	44	42	41	40	39	38	37	36
136 (300)																	50	48	47	45	44	43	42	41	40	39	38	37

A. Guidelines for adolescent preventive services (GAPS)
American Medical Association

Recognizing today's crisis in adolescent health, the American Medical Association is recommending a fundamental change in health care, aimed at prevention. To deal with the health crisis, AMA has developed the Guidelines for Adolescent Preventive Services (GAPS), which calls for doctors to screen their teenage patients each year for major health problems, including weight and eating problems.

This is an approach that can fit well into the new unified health paradigm dealing with weight and eating issues. For now the GAPS program focuses on the screening and evaluation phase. Later this will be followed by the second phase providing more specific recommendations on prevention and treatment.

The GAPS program recommendations that relate to weight and eating are as follows:

■ All adolescents (age 11-21) should be screened during annual health visits for eating disorders and obesity. This includes height and weight measures and questioning about body image and dieting patterns.

■ Adolescents should be assessed for organic disease, anorexia nervosa, or bulimia if any of the following are found: weight loss of more than 10 percent of the previous year; recurrent dieting when not overweight; use of self-induced emesis, laxatives, starvation, or diuretics to lose weight; distorted body image; or body mass index (BMI) below the 5th percentile.

■ Adolescents with a BMI equal to or greater than the 95th percentile are overweight and should have an in-depth dietary and health assessment to determine psychosocial morbidity and risk for future cardiovascular disease.

■ Adolescents with a BMI between the 85th and 94th percentile are at risk for becoming overweight. A dietary and health assessment to determine psychosocial morbidity and risk for future cardiovascular disease should be performed on these youth if:
  ● their BMI has increased by two or more units during the previous 12 months;
  ● there is a family history of premature heart disease, obesity, hypertension, or diabetes mellitus;
  ● they express concern about their weight;
  ● they have elevated serum cholesterol levels or blood pressure.

■ If this assessment is negative, these adolescents should be provided general dietary and exercise counseling and should be monitored annually.

Three times, during early, middle and late adolescence, the doctor or other provider is advised to perform a comprehensive physical examination. At least twice during their child's adolescence, it is recommended that all parents receive education about adolescent health care.

AMA calls the GAPS program a major change from the traditional approach to adolescent health care, which focused on and treated specific medical problems alone. The new emphasis is on comprehensive assessment and early detection of health problems. The annual visits offer an opportunity to provide health education and develop a therapeutic relationship. The health provider also plays an important role in coordinating adolescent health promotion by complementing the guidance received from family, school and community, whereas in the past it was considered to be independent. AMA offers physician training on how to deliver these kinds of preventive services.

According to the 1995 GAPS Recommendations Monograph:

"Changes in adolescent morbidity and mortality during the past several decades have created a health crisis for today's youth. Unintended pregnancy, STDs, alcohol and drug abuse, and eating disorders are just some of the health problems faced by an increasing number of adolescents from all sectors of society.

"This health crisis requires a fundamental change in the emphasis of adolescent services. School and community organizations have responded to the need for change by increasing health education programming. Primary care physicians and other health providers must respond by making preventive services a greater component of their clinical practice."

Thus the stage is ideally set for the AMA to introduce physicians to the united health approach. It is critical that wise decisions be made before issuing the upcoming AMA recommendations on treatment of weight and eating problems, to avoid further harm to young people and to advance the goal of healthy children of all sizes.

GAPS screening resources include:

- AMA Guidelines for Adolescent Preventive Services: Recommendations and Rationale

- Clinical Evaluation and Management Handbook

- Implementation and Resource Manual

- Implementation Training Workshop

- GAPS Presentation Kit

Information and materials available from:

Department of Adolescent Health
American Medical Association
515 North State Street
Chicago, IL 60610
(312-464-5570; fax 312-464-5842)

B. Working with teenagers

Teens & Diets: No Weigh
How to deliver the nondieting message
by Linda Omichinski, RD

The importance of breaking the diet cycle at an early age can't be overemphasized. As health professionals we can take some new directions and responsibility to change the cultural message.

What legacy are we passing on to the next generation? Are we a society of dieters unhappy with the way we look because media messages tell us we should be slim? Food preoccupation and dieting has become an obsession for too many. The right to enjoy food and accept the inherent satisfaction and sustainment that comes from nourishing your body seems to have been stolen away.

The good news is that healthy, nondieting is a valid lifestyle choice that comes with a freeing set of parameters and characteristics far surpassing the restrictions of a diet lifestyle. There is no better time for establishing a new way of living than the teen years.

Part of working with teens involves letting go of the control and enabling them to make the decisions. Comments like, "That's a very interesting point of view. Could you tell me more about that?" lets teens express their own perspective.

Empowerment techniques are ideally suited for teen development.

It's critical to have an open attitude about the seeming negatives in this age group so that true learning can take place. Personal qualities of openness, caring and a good sense of humor aid educators of any age group and particularly for teens.

Build a relationship based on trust; share personal stories and some background so they can identify with you. Treat teens as adults, with the acceptance that will enable feeling good, relaxing and opening up to occur. Emphasize that no question is stupid. Use lots of humor.

We recommend four prongs to reach the public with a nondieting health message for teens: through schools, teen grapevines, parental concern, and the medical and health professional community.

On the following pages are empowerment techniques and program goals for the teen and family as advocated by the Teens & Diets: No Weigh program. Reprinted with permission from the HUGS teen facilitator package Teens & Diets: No Weigh, by Linda Omichinski, Copyright 1995. HUGS International Inc., Box 102A, RR#3, Portage la Prairie, Manitoba, R1N 3A3, Canada (1-800-565-4847).

How to enable teen powered health decisions

Facilitated empowerment techniques

Empowerment technique	Offsets or counteracts	Positive outcomes	Teen examples	Facilitator guidance/comment
1. Interactive listening: you want to hear back the message the teen received from you.	Preaching.	Teen will listen better when his feedback is seen to be important to you, ensuring that important concepts/facts are more likely to be retained.	*"I don't eat bread or pasta because it makes me feel fat."*	Could you tell me what you mean by feeling fat? Do you mean your jeans are feeling tight? Do you mean you are feeling puffy? Let's explore why eating more carbohydrates like bread or pasta makes you feel this way.
2. Consistent discovery and emphasis of the positive.	Self-absorption and perceived negatives about personal appearance.	A broadening of the teen's thinking pattern. There are reasons for the way things are that can't be changed. Some things have to be accepted.	*"I hate my skinny legs."*	That's your natural, genetic body shape. Look at your broad shoulders. You must look fabulous in a halter top.
3. Present a process for decisionmaking: study, reflect, decide.	Should and must orders.	A set of rules is fine for a game, but for your whole life? Teen appreciates range of choice in many situations.	*"My Mom says I have to eat fruit for dessert at each meal."*	Suggest to your mom that having your "mealtime" fruit after school and before supper when you're really hungry works better for you.
4. Make stories and content relevant to teen lifestyle.	Didactic teaching.	When the teen can truly put themselves in the situation, they are more likely to remember the facts and scenario.	*"All the cool kids smoke; I'm going to start so I can be part of that group."*	Cool kids also like computers. You can really impress people with what you're doing on the Internet. What about making your own group?

Empowerment technique	Offsets or counteracts	Positive outcomes	Teen examples	Facilitator guidance/comment
5. Encouragement of self-awareness and self identity.	Compliance expectations.	The teen understands uniqueness as a strength and often marvels at the diversity of her character and range	"I hate volleyball. Why is that the only sport that means anything in this school?"	Fine; it's not for everyone. Let's see what you would like to do.
6. Affirm failures as necessary to growth & discover better ways; redefine failure; redefine success	"Failure is an end result" thinking	Teen begins to see the two sides of the same coin perspective in all issues.	"I'm still pigging out after school, even though I know better."	You are working on the right pattern for you. It takes time to figure out what will really work. You're very successful at being aware of what you're doing; that's the first step.
7. Support and acknowledge personal decisions that have been made. Decisions don't always lead to action but can be the choice not to participate. The key is that a process of examination has taken place.	Issuing approval or disapproval about decisions	Teen begins to see that experimentation & action is much preferable to drifting & letting others make the choices that affect them.	"Guess what — I decided not to take swimming lessons with my best friend."	That's an interesting choice if you've always done things together. You must have another interest in mind or maybe you just want a break from lessons. Sometimes it's harder to decide to stop doing something instead of starting something. Could you tell me more about how you decided?
8. Point out weight and diet & body shape bias.	The perfect body/ perfect weight syndrome.	A broader view & enhanced critical thinking; teens sees that society has a problem with unrealistic standards & norms; it's not just her or her family.	"I saw on TV last night that Terri Hatcher of Lois & Clark might have an eating disorder. She looked great before & now even her neck bones stick out. I heard she just eats one plate of broccoli each day."	What kind of standards do we buy into? This is the model that supported the development of the concepts in Building the Road to Healthier Living ...teen powered health decisions.

Teens & Diets: No Weigh

Program goals
- Establish a lifestyle perspective for young people to take responsibility for their own food needs and activities.
- Enable teens to take responsibility for their eating preferences.
- Help teens understand and incorporate into their own lives the interconnectedness of food, activity and attitude.
- Provide knowledge, instill skills and build confidence so that young people are equipped to find their personal balance of food and physical activity to energize their lifestyle choices.
- Involve the family unit in the process of understanding the necessity for individual patterns of nourishment.
- Provide information about body image and self-esteem.
- Provide new knowledge about food.
- Provide new knowledge about physical activity.
- Demonstrate how to be experimental and assertive.

For the teen
- How to take responsibility for own appetite and tastes within the family setting.
- How to understand signals in own body for hunger.
- How to use consistent physical activity as a source of energy.
- How to eat for energy and health.
- How to appreciate genetic and growth factors in personal appearance changes.
- How to have a healthier body image.
- How to express oneself assertively.
- How to critically look at media messages around health/body image.
- How to measure health as a state of energetic and confident well-being as opposed to a number on the scale.

For the family
- Respect individual food preferences.
- Offer a variety of foods.
- Understand physical differences in the need for food.
- Convey non-judgmental attitudes.
- Demonstrate unreserved acceptance of the teen.

From the HUGS for Teens program, Teens & Diets: No Weigh, Building the road to healthier living, 1995, by Linda Omichinski, RD.

C. Radical animal rights agenda
"Very dangerous for kids."

Radical animal rights groups are coming into American schools and spreading a message that is undermining the health of our children, usually under the guise of teaching about animals or endangered species, or saving the environment. While "animal learn" sounds harmless enough, the real goal of these groups appears to be to persuade children to stop consuming animal foods of any kind, even milk, and to turn kids into vegans, the most restrictive type of vegetarian.

Many children are traumatized by what they see in the graphic videos shown by these groups. This is not education, it is proselytizing in the schools. Parents trust schools to teach their children in balanced, objective ways, and often have no idea what is happening, until too late. Schools do not sensationalize cruel or deadly acts against humans in war or criminality (imagine the terror they would engender if they did). Yet, even administrators and school boards inadvertently play into the hands of these groups. The mystery is, why do teachers invite or allow these animal rights speakers into their classrooms?

Our children are being seduced in great numbers by these fanatical Pied Pipers. It's one of the nation's fastest growing social crusades and last year pulled in over $300 million from a membership of about 10 million, up more than 400 percent in the last decade, according to Sally Satel, Yale University School of Medicine.

Below are reports from responsible leaders about the harm these groups are doing.

"Self appointed "nutritionists" should not be allowed to go into the schools to present an emotional diatribe about society's shortcomings in the areas of nutrition, air, soil, water and animal cruelty, place blame on certain groups, and then irresponsibly teach the new vegan diet pattern, leaving some inadequate brochures behind. The children will go home short on facts and long on anger. We do not believe in setting children up for this emotional confrontation with their families.

"The gross treatment of animals as shown on the EarthSave video in schools is emotional blackmail. Farmers could not stay in business by treating animals inhumanely — they would not grow properly or would die of sickness. Why not attack a perceived problem directly by reporting to authorities, instead of by the passive self-denial of not eating veal?" — *Nancy Tullis, RD   Chair, Reliable Nutrition Information, Louisville Dietetic Association, Louisville, Ky.*

"The dangerous campaign being waged by animal-rights activists is not a struggle against medical science alone; it is a struggle against humanity."
—*Seattle Times, Sept. 11, 1989*

"There is a sense that these kids have been traumatized . . . influenced by the message that the animal rights people are taking into the schools. They are trying to eat perfectly, and they get this black and white sense of what is perfect: 'If I'm a nice person I'll be a vegetarian, and if I'm not a nice person I'll eat meat." — *Monika Woolsey, MS, RD, Eating Disorder Specialist, Glendale, Ariz*

"Major groups such as PETA have found big success in attracting young members, after-school animal-rights clubs have sprung up across the country, and the Dissection Hotline set up to counsel students has received 40,000 calls in three years, says its director, Pat Graham.

"Part of the reason for the youth explosion is PETA's success at making animal rights a hip cause. In addition to school mailings, teens have flocked to the movement after seeing endorsements by movie stars. PETA also sets up tables at concerts by such groups as Guns N' Roses.

"High schoolers aren't the only new advocates, either. Nearly 5,000 subscribers under age 10 receive a magazine called PETA Kids, featuring cartoons and connect-the-dots puzzles, along with advice on how to become a vegetarian and how to prevent animal cruelty." — *Wall Street Journal Sept. 2, 1992.*

"We are an animal loving nation, and so it should come as no surprise that as children who have been devoted to their dogs, cats and hamsters grow older, they become highly supportive of efforts to protect animal species that are endangered. The scientific and medical communities probably will be alarmed, however, to discover that according to the findings of the most recent Gallup Youth Survey, a majority of the nation's teenagers also say they support the "animal rights movement," even if it would mean the end to laboratory and medical tests that use animals.

"A plurality of 41 percent support the movement very much, and are joined by 26 percent who say they are somewhat in favor of it. Among the remaining teens, 18 percent say they are somewhat opposed to animal rights, 14 percent are very much opposed, and 3 percent have no opinion about the movement . . . As teens grow older their support diminishes somewhat." — *George Gallup, Jr., and Alec Gallup, The Gallup Youth Survey, 1991*

"This is very dangerous for kids . . . Because they consider themselves morally superior, many vegetarians exhibit no reservations against using mind-control techniques or terrorism to actualize their agenda. Mind control includes using information selectively to 'educate.' It may also include traumatizing people emotionally to condition them against the use of animal foods . . . As a religion, vegetarianism attracts the guilt-ridden. And it seduces the unskeptical by causing guilt and/or by instilling false guilt. Guilt leads to self-denial." — *Willliam Jarvis, PhD, president of the National Council Against Health Fraud*

"The other day I attended a religious revival . . . the local meeting of the Progressive Animal Welfare Society (PAWS). Members of the latest, fastest-growing, and most politically correct religion on the block — the religion of animal rights. I knew that animal-rights activists existed, but I never thought they were important — just some people who, if ignored long enough, would fade away.

Attendance at a single PAWS meeting proved me wrong.

"I sat through the meeting in a state of shock. The information fed to the audience was so exaggerated, misinformed, inflammatory, and sometimes so wrong that I kept wondering if it were some kind of joke — but the people in the audience believed every word. They are in a holy mission of intimidation and misinformation to spread the Truth. And, in the environmentally sensitive culture we have now, the message is spreading. Animal rights are becoming the 'hot new issue of the '90s.'

". . . The money you send for PAWS' low-cost neutering clinics might be used to shut down a research laboratory that could find a cure for AIDS. The money you send to stop fur trapping might be used in the campaign against research in brain injuries." —*Michael Kerr, Seattle Times, May 1, 1991*

"Animal rights advocates (at least the leaders) are the ones who are anti-life; their hatred of man is openly and loudly proclaimed. They must be fought and stopped in the name of morality." *— Edwin Locke, PhD, College of Business and Management, University of Maryland, College Park, MD.*

Medical research threatened

"A humane concern for the welfare of animals means wanting to see that they are treated without cruelty, are properly cared for and not made to suffer unnecessary pain. That's right and good. But that is quite unlike the fanaticism of the animal rights extremists. Some of these extremists . . . have vandalized labs, set them on fire, destroyed research files, harassed scientists and technicians, and issued death threats.

"Alex Pacheco, one of PETA's founders, has said that, 'Arson, property destruction, burglary or theft are acceptable crimes when they directly alleviate the pain and suffering of an animal.'

"Ingrid Newkirk heads People for the Ethical Treatment of Animals, or PETA . . . one of perhaps more than 400 such animal rights organizations across the country. She once said on a radio talk show that morally there is no basic difference between human beings and other animals, 'A rat is a pig is a dog is a boy.'

"Virtually all medical advances in the 20th century have required laboratory animal research, including vaccines for polio and measles, cancer chemotherapy, open heart surgery, and insulin for diabetics." *— American Medical Association*

"Biomedical research is essential to the health and well-being of every person in our society. Advances have dramatically improved the quality and prolonged the duration of life throughout the world.

"However, the ability of the scientific community to continue its efforts to improve personal and public health is being threatened by a movement to eliminate the use of animals. This movement is spearheaded by groups of radical animal rights activists whose views are far outside mainstream public attitudes and whose tactics range from sophisticated lobbying, fund raising, propaganda and misinformation campaigns to violent attacks on research facilities and individual scientists.

"The magnitude of violent animal rights activities is staggering. In the U.S.

alone, since 1980, animal rights groups have staged more than 29 raids on U.S. research facilities, stealing over 2,000 animals, causing more than 7 million dollars in physical damages and ruining years of scientific research. Animal activist groups have engaged in similar activities in Great Britain, Western Europe, Canada and Australia. Various groups in these countries have claimed responsibility for the bombing of cars, institutions, stores, and the private homes of researchers." — *World Medical Association Statement, France, 1989.*

Equating humans with animals

"**It seems to me you can't argue** that human beings are morally the same as animals, and then also argue that we should behave differently toward animals than they behave toward each other — or us, given the chance.

"Nature is beautiful, but it is also harsh. To survive, most organisms eat other organisms, either plant or animal. And there are many places in the world where careless humans still become dinner for tigers, sharks, crocodiles, piranha and other predators. I doubt if they worry much about the morality of eating a human being.

"The fact is, we are the only species that does worry about these things. Besides our complex languages, our free will and our reason, we are the only animals with a moral sensibility — and that does set us apart. In fact, that's why we care about the humane treatment of animals . . . (but) polls show that the American public overwhelmingly rejects the activists' claim that there is no difference between animals and humans." — *American Medical Association*

"**Ingrid Newkirk has equated the death of chickens** with the deaths of people who died in concentration camps during World War II. The idea of animal rights may set out to insure that animals are treated as human beings, but by blurring the essential distinction between the two, it lends itself just as readily to the suggestion that human beings may be treated as animals. And given the history of the twentieth century and the sufferings of millions around the world, there is clear danger that the latter interpretation will enjoy ascendancy. Thus the doctrine that purports to elevate the status of all living things is, in the end, a doctrine that debases the status of mankind, and endangers our essential freedoms." — *Constance Horner, U.S. Under Secretary of Health and Human Services, 1990*

"**These folks routinely compare scientists** to Nazis . . . Yet Hitler, too . . . thought it better to experiment on humans . . . like the animal rights advocates . . . There are similarities . . . The attitude toward crippled children, for instance, and the ethics of human experimentation. In the first place, Adolf Hitler himself was an animal "rights" person and a vegetarian. This is a fact. Goebels promised on a variety of public occasions that one feature of the Third Reich would be a new respect for animals, and a phasing out of animal experimentation.

"At the same time the Nazi party was busy anthropomorphizing animals it was also at work dehumanizing people who were not up to what was considered par, physically and mentally. Listen closely to the words of animal rights advocates. Do you detect the dehumanization of certain groups?

What do animal rights activists want?
American Medical Association

Agenda of the animal "rights" movement:
- Elimination of animals in research
- No meat, dairy products
- No leather, silk
- No zoos, circuses, aquariums
- No pets

Tactics of some animal "rights" groups:
- Public disinformation campaign
- Arson
- Destruction of medical research laboratories, offices, files
- Bombings
- Harassment
- Death threats

Instead of all this, *animal welfare* concerns are for responsible care of animals, preventing cruelty, and support for neutering and adoption.

"Read Peter Singer's latest book, 'Should the Baby Live? The Problem of Handicapped Infants.' He's the Australian philosopher who wrote 'Animal Liberation'." — *Jon Franklin, Professor of Journalism, University of Oregon, Eugene*

NOTE TO THE MEDIA:

Writers, editors and producers need to be aware of their potential manipulation by animal rights activists, and the "political correctness" that the media has accorded them. For example, the press recently attacked a teenage boy with an incurable illness whose *Make-a-Wish* was to hunt big game in Alaska. Instead of destroying the dreams of a young boy, as they seemed determined to do, journalists would better have reported on the source of these attacks. At the very least, they can ignore them. Loving and caring for animals is very different from the chilling radical animal rights agenda, and this needs to be reported.

"The AMA continues to marvel at how effectively a fringe organization of questionable repute continues to hoodwink the media," says the American Medical Association. The AMA maintains a press office at its headquarters in Chicago that will answer media questions on animal rights issues (312-464-5382; fax 312-464-2450).

D. Dysfunctional eating
Research basis

Among the important sources on which the concept of dysfunctional eating is developed are: the early work on restrained eating by Janet Polivy and Peter Herman[1]; writings and presentations by Susan Wooley[2]; writings and work by Ellyn Satter on normal eating and her workshops on "Treating the dieting casualty"[3]; Linda Omichinski's nondiet leadership and program development devoted to breaking the dieting cycle[4]; the concept development on thinking about food by Dan and Kim Reiff[5]; starvation studies, including the Minnesota Experiment,[6] United Nations reports on world malnutrition,[7] and Colin Turnbull's striking portrait of *The Mountain People*[8]; national and local studies showing the high prevalence of dieting and disordered eating among children and adolescents[9]; eating disorder research showing mental and physical effects of eating disorders, and the associations of eating disorders with dieting[10]; discussions on the risks of dieting and the need to treat chronic dieting syndrome by Arnold Andersen and Mike Bowers[11]; and the progress of No Diet Day observances, led by Mary Evans Young,[12] and Eating Disorder Awareness Week, organized by eating disorder specialists.[13]

Most of this information has been reviewed in *Healthy Weight Journal* over the past 11 years, and is discussed extensively and referenced in the book *Health Risks of Weight Loss*.[14]

1. Herman P, J Polivy. A boundary model for the regulation of eating. Eating and its disorders, edit Stunkard and Steller, 1984, 141-56. Raven Press, N.Y.
   Healthy Weight J Mar/Apr 1996;10:2:32-33.
2. Wooley S, W Wooley. Should obesity be treated at all? Eating and its Disorders, Stunkard and Steller, edits; 1984. Raven Press, N.Y.
3. Satter, Ellyn, How to get your kids to eat — but not too much, Bull Publ, Palo Alto, Calif.
   Workshops, "Treating the dieting casualty," Satter Assoc., Madison, Wis.
4. Omichinski L, You Count, Calories Don't, 1992; HUGS facilitator programs, HUGS International, Box 102A, Rt 3, Portage la Prairie, Manitoba, R1N 3A3, Canada; Teens & Diets — No Weigh, Healthy Weight J 1996;10:3:49-52; Berg F, Nondiet movement gains strength HWJ/Obesity & Health Sep/Oct 1992;6:5:82-90.
5. Reiff D, KK Lampson Reiff, Eating Disorders: Nutrition Therapy in the Recovery Process, 1992. Aspen, Gaithersburg, MD; Personal communication with Dan Reiff, 1996.
6. Keys A, et al. Biology of human starvation, 1950. U of Minn Press, Minneapolis, Minn.
   Berg F, Starvation stages in weight loss patients similar to famine victims, HWJ/Obesity & Health Apr 1989;3:4:27-30.

7. Body Mass Index. FAO, A measure of chronic energy deficiency in adults, 1994, United Nations report.

    Berg F, World starvation: weight may be best tool to measure malnutrition, Healthy Weight J May/Jun 1995;9:3:47-49.

8. Turnbull, Colin, 1972, The Mountain People. Simon and Schuster, N.Y.

9. CDC USHHS, Behavioral Risk Survey; Calorie Control Council, 1991 National Survey.

    Berg F, Who is dieting in the U.S. Healthy Weight Journal/Obesity & Health 1992;6:3:48-49.

    Dieting and purging behavior in black and white high school students, JADA 1992;92:3:306-312.

    Adolescents dieting; JAMA 1991;266:2811-2812.

    Berg F, Harmful weight loss practices among adolescents, HWJ/O&H Jul/Aug 1992;6:4:69-72.

10. Fallon P, Katzman M, Wooley S, Feminist perspectives on eating disorders 1994, Guilford Press, N.Y.

    Baker D, R Sansone, Overview of eating disorders, 1994:1-10, NEDO.

    Kaplan A, P Garfinkel, Medical issues and the eating disorders, 1993, Brunner/Mazel, N.Y.

    Berg F, Eating disorders: physical and mental effects, Healthy Weight J Mar/Apr 1995;9:2:27-30.

    Smolak L, M Levine, Toward an empirical basis for primary prevention of eating problems with elementary school children, Eat Disorders 1994;2:4:293-307

11. Andersen A. The last word, Eating Disorders 1994;2:1:81-82.

    Bowers M. The last word. Eating Disorders 1994;2:4:375-377.

12. Young, Mary Evans, Diet Breaking, 1996, Hodder & Stoughton, London.

13. Biely J, Eating Disorder Awareness Week '96, EDAP Matters Winter 1996;2.

14. Berg F. Health Risks of Weight Loss, 1995. Chapter 1. General treatment risks, 14-26; Ch 7. Eating disorders, 56-62; Ch 8. Psychological risks, 63-69; Ch 9. Weight cycling, 70-79; Ch 11. Thinness: a cultural obsession, 89-99; Ch 13. To treat or not to treat, 108-113. 66:2811-2812; Berg F, Harmful weight loss practices among adolescents, HWJ/O&H Jul/Aug 1992;6:4:69.

E. Child-centered resources
The health approach

How to get your Kid to Eat — But not too much, by Ellyn Satter. Birth through adolescence, 1987, softcover, 396 pages. Bull Publishing, Box 208, Palo Alto, CA 94302 (415-322-2855).

Child of Mine — Feeding with love and good sense, by Ellyn Satter. Pregnancy through toddler stage, 1983, softcover. Bull Publishing.

Feeding with Love and Good Sense, by Ellyn Satter. Series of four 15-minute videotapes about feeding the infant, older baby, toddler and preschooler, set of four on one tape. Ellyn Satter Associates, 4226 Mandan Crescent, Madison, WI 53711 (1-800-808-7976; fax 608-271-7976).

Feeding with Love and Good Sense Training Manual, 103 pages, reproducable teaching materials. **Ellyn Satter's Vision workshop**. Ellyn Satter Assoc.,

Teens & Diets — No Weigh: Building the road to healthier living. HUGS for Teens program franchised to licensed health professionals, by Linda Omichinski, RD. Eight lesson plans, scripts and resources. Supported with newsletter, teen journal, parent guidebook, 1995. HUGS International, Box 102A, RR3, Portage la Prairie, Manitoba, Canada R1N 3A3 (204-428-3432; 1-800-565-4847; fax 204-428-5072).

Vitality Leader's Kit. Contains Vitality health promotion materials that focus on a fundamental shift from treatment to prevention of weight problems including overweight, underweight, eating disorders, weight preoccupation and negative body image, 1994. Health Services and Promotion, Health and Welfare Canada, 4th Floor, Jeanne Mance Bldg., Ottawa, Ontario, Canada K1A 1B4 (613-957-8331; fax 613-941-2399).

Solving your Child's Eating Problems, by Jane Hirschmann and Lela Zaphiropoulos. 1985. Fawcett Columbine/Ballantine, New York.

Eating disorder resources

Girls in the 90s. Sandra Susan Friedman, BA, BSW, MA. Eating disorders preventive program for pre- and early-adolescent girls. Open-ended groups, 10-12 weeks. Developed in British Columbia for the Boundary Health Unit. Salal Books, Box 309, 101-1184 Denman St., Vancouver, BC, Canada V6G 2M9 (604-689-8399).

Discovery of Dawn. Video. Causes, symptoms and effects of eating disorders organized around story of survivor. For rent or purchase. University of Wisconsin-Green Bay, WI 54311 (1-800-633-7445; fax 414-465-2576; newist@uwgb.edu).

Eating disorder organizations; these groups have information, newsletters, videos and brochures available:

EDAP. Eating Disorders Awareness and Prevention. Sponsors Eating Disorder Awareness Week (2nd week

Feb.), puppet show. 603 Stewart St., #803, Seattle, WA 98101 (206-382-3587; fax 206-382-4793).

ANAD. Association of Anorexia Nervosa and Associated Disorders, PO Box 7, Highland Park, IL 60035 (847-831-3438).

ANRED. Anorexia Nervosa and Related Disorders. PO Box 5102, Eugene OR 97405 (503-344-1144).

NEDO. National Eating Disorders Organization. 6655 S. Yale Ave., Tulsa, OK 74136.

Academy for Eating Disorders. Div. Adol. Medicine, Montefiore Medical Center, 111 E 210th St. Bronx, NY 10467 (718-920-6782; fax 718-920-5289).

National Eating Disorder Information Centre. College Wing 1-211, 200 Elizabeth St., Toronto ON M5G 2C4, Canada (416-340-4156; fax 416-340-4736).

Gurze catalog. Specializes in eating disorder books. Gurze Books, PO Box 2238, Carlsbad, CA 92018 (1-800-756-7533, www.gurze.com).

Helping large children

Am I Fat? Helping Young Children Accept Differences in Body Size, by Joanne Ikeda, MA, RD, and Priscilla Naworski, MS, CHES. Softcover, 110 pages. ETR Associates, PO Box 1830, Santa Cruz, CA 95061-1880 (1-800-321-4407).

If My Child is Too Fat, What should I do about it? Booklet for parents by Joanne Ikeda (501-642-2790; fax 510-642-0535).

Children and Weight: What's a parent to do? and **Family Choices for Good Health.** Low-literacy booklets for parents by Joanne Ikeda and Rita

Mitchell. ANR Publications, University of California, 6701 San Pablo Ave., Oakland, CA 94608 (415-642-2431).

Children and Weight: What's a parent to do? 12-minute videotape, includes sample parent books. English and Spanish. Visual Media, 1441 Research Park Drive, University of California, Davis, CA 95616.

Kid's Project, Packet of size acceptance materials. Kids Come in all Sizes workshops. Council on Size & Weight Discrimination, Miriam Berg, P.O. Box 305, Mt. Marion, NY 12456 (914-679-1209; fax 914-679-1206).

Good News for Big Kids. National Association to Advance Fat Acceptance. Pamphlet. NAAFA, PO Box 188620, Sacramento, CA 95818 (1-800-442-1214; 916-558-6880; fax 916-558-6881).

Size acceptance resources with some information on children or teens.

Size Wise, by Judy Sullivan. 1997. Avon Books, 1350 Ave. of Americas, New York, NY 10019.

Radiance magazine, PO Box 31703, Oakland CA 94604.

Big Beautiful Woman magazine, 8484 Wilshire Blvd, #900, Beverly Hills, CA 90211.

References

Chapter 1

1. Berg F. Harmful weight loss practices widespread among adolescents. HWJ/Obesity & Health 1992;6:4:69-72.
2. P.L.E.A.S.E. Newsl. Spring-Summer 1996;2.
3. Third report on nutrition monitoring in the US, Vol 1-2, Dec 1995. National Center for Health Statistics, NHANES III. Life Sciences Research Office, Interagency Board for Nutrition Monitoring and Related Research, US Dept of Health and Human Services, US Dept of Agriculture.
   Natl Ctr for Health Statistics, NHANES III. Advance Data Nov 14, 1994.
4. Youth Risk Behavior Surveillance — US, 1995. Morbidity and Mortality Weekly Report, CDC, US Public Health Service. Sept 27, 1996:45:SS-4.
   JAMA 1991;266:2811-12.
5. Vitality Leader's Kit, 1994. Health Services and Promotion, Health and Welfare Canada. 4th Floor, Jeanne Mance Bldg, Ottawa, Ontario, Canada K1A 1B4 (613-957-8331).
6. JAMA 1996;276:1907-1915.
   Berg F. Task Force advises against diet drugs. Healthy Weight Journal 1997;11:2:27.
7. The Dietary Guidelines for Americans, 4th Edition, 1995. Consumer Information Center, Pueblo, CO.
8. Berg F. New guidelines given for "healthy weight." Healthy Weight J. May/Jun 1996;10:3:44, 53-54, 57.
9. Choosing a safe and successful weight-loss program, WIN, NIDDK.
10. National Task Force on the Prevention and Treatment of Obesity. Weight Cycling. JAMA 1994;272;15:11696-1202.
11. Berg F. Weight loss campaign heats up. 1995;9:1:4, 11-12, 18-19.
12. Weighing the Options. 1995, Natl Academy Press, Wash., DC.
13. Berg F. Review: Weighing the Options. Healthy Weight J. May/Jun 1995;9:3:57-58.
14. NIH Technology Assessment Conference: Methods for Voluntary weight loss and control. 1992. Office of Medical Applic. Research, NIH, Federal Bldg., Rm 618, Bethesda, MD 20892.

Chapter 2

1. Pipher M. Reviving Ophelia. 1994.

Ballantine Books, Random House, NY.
2. Fallon P, M Katzman, S Wooley, edits. Feminist perspectives on eating disorders. 1994. Guilford Press, NY.
   Berg F. Health Risks of Weight Loss, 1995;89. Healthy Weight J, Hettinger, ND.
3. Newsweek. Feb 1, 1993, 64-65.
   Berg F. Gaunt idols. Healthy Weight J./Obesity & Health Mar/Apr 1993;7:2:23.
4. Eating Disorders 1993;1:1:52-61.
   Berg F. Television ads promote dieting. HWJ/Obesity & Health Nov/Dec 1993;7:6:106.
5. Kilbourne J. Still killing us softly: Advertising and the obsession with thinness. Fallon, see 2.
6. Wolf N. The beauty myth: how images of beauty are used against women, 1991. Morrow, NY.
7. I J Eating Disorders 1992; 11:1:85-89.
8. Berg F. Thin mania turns up pressure. HWJ/Obesity & Health Sep/Oct 1992;6:5:83.
9. Berg F. Health Risks of Weight Loss, 1995;90. Healthy Weight J., ND.
10. Morgan L. Why are girls obsessed with their weight? Seventeen Nov. 1989;118-119, 145, 150, 154.
11. Reported from New Scientist by Am Anorexia/Bulimia Assoc Newsletter Spring 1994;8.
    Berg F. Health Risks of Weight Loss, 1995;92. Healthy Weight J., ND.
12. Oswalt R, J Davis. Societal influences on a thinner body size in children. Proceedings and abstracts of the annual meeting of the Eastern Psychological Association. Philadelphia, PA. April 1990.
13. Eating Disorder Awareness Week Kit: Celebrating our natural sizes. 1996, National Eating Disorder Information Centre, Toronto.
14. Eating Disorders 1993;1:2:109-114.
    Berg F. False media messages. HWJ/Obesity & Health Jan/Feb 1994;8:1:5.
15. Nutr Forum Sep/Oct 1989, from Pediatrics 1989 83:393-397.
    Berg F. Weight Terror. HWJ/Obesity & Health Jan 1990;4:1:1.
16. Morgan L. Why are girls obsessed with their weight? Seventeen Nov. 1989;118-119, 145, 150, 154.
17. Grange D, J Tibbs, J Selibowitz. Eating attitudes, body shape, and self-disclosure in a community sample of adolescent girls and

boys. Eating Dis 1995:3:3:253-264.

18. Crisp A. Anorexia nervosa in a young male. In Treating Eating Disorders, J Werne, edit. 1996:6. Jossey-Bass Inc, San Francisco.

19. Smolak L, M Levine. Toward an empirical basis for primary prevention of eating problems with elementary school children. Eat Disorders 1994;2:4:293-307.

20. Food Nutr News 1993;65:1:4.
Berg, HRWL, *see 9:92.*

21. Gustafson-Larson, AM, RD Terry. Weight-related behaviors and concerns of fourth-grade children. J of the Am Dietetic Assoc 1992:818-822.

22. Nichter M, S Park, M Nichter, Body image and weight concerns among African American and white adolescent females. Anthro. Dept, U of Arizona, Tucson, AZ.
Berg F. Beauty ideas are fluid. Healthy Weight J., Mar/Apr 1995;9:2:26.
Berg, HRWL, *see 9:123.*

23. Young, Mary Evans. Diet Breaking: Having it all without having to diet. Hodder and Stoughton. London. 1995:5-9.

24. Rothblum E. I'll die for the revolution but don't ask me not to diet. 1994;53-76.
Fallon, *see 2.*
Berg, *see 9: 91.*

25. Berg F. Girls and dolls. Healthy Weight J. 1997;11:1:6.

26. Meletiche. NAAFA News Sept/Oct 1991:5. Meletiche L. Barbie: Symbol of oppression. HWJ/Obesity & Health Sep/Oct 1993;7:5:96.

27. Smolak L, M Levine. The role of parents in the prevention of disordered eating. NEDO Newsletter 1994;17:3:1-9.

28. Levine P. President's message. Eating Disorders Awareness and Prevention Newsletter. Spring 1995:1-3.

29. Tolman D, E Debold. Conflicts of body and image, 301-317. Fallon, *see 2.*

30. Larkin J, C Rice and V Russell. Slipping through the cracks: sexual harassment, eating problems, and the problem of embodiment. Eat Disorders 1996;4:1:5-26.

31. Levine P. The Last Word. Eat Disorders 1995;3:1:92-95.

Chapter 3

1. Niven C, D Carroll. The Health psychology of women. Harwood Academic Publ., Chur, Switzerland. 1993:115.

2. Berg F. Kids fear being fat early. HWJ/Obesity & Health May/June 1993;7:3:46-47. JADA 1992;92;92:7:851-53.

3. Reiff D, KK Lampson Reiff, Eating Disorders: Nutrition Therapy in the Recovery Process, 1992. Aspen, Gaithersburg, MD;

Personal communication, D. Reiff, 1996.

4. Keys, Ancel et al. The Biology of Human Starvation. School of Public Health, 1950. U of Minnesota Press, Minneapolis, MN.

5. Estes L, M Crago, C Shisslak. Eating disorders prevention. The Renfrew Perspective, 1996;2:1:3-5.
Fallon, *see Ch2:2.*
Berg, *see 2.*

6. Smolak, *see Ch2:19.*

7. Fallon, *see Ch2:2.*

8. Turnbull, Colin. The Mountain People. 1972, Simon and Schuster, NY

9. Restaurants USA 1994;14:18-21.
Berg, F. Customers want bigger meals Healthy Weight Journal Mar/Apr 1995;9:2:26.

10. Taste, Health, and the Social Meal. Special issue. J. of Gastronomy. Winter/Sp 1993.
Berg F. Review of special issue, J Gastronomy. Healthy Weight J., May/Jun 1994;8:3:59.

11. Satter, Ellyn. How to Get Your Kid to Eat . . . But Not Too Much, 1987; Child of Mine: Feeding With Love and Good Sense, 1983. Bull Publishing, Palo Alto, CA.

12. HUGS Club News, Jan. 1997, p6.

13. Berg F. Weight-loss programs for children and adolescents. HWJ/Obesity & Health Oct 1989;3:10:78.
Nutrition News 1988;51:2:5-7.

Chapter 4

1. Alexander-Mott L, DB Lumsden. Understanding Eating Disorders. Taylor & Francis, Washington, DC 1994:290.

2. Reiff, *see Ch3:3,* p312.

3. Eating Disorder Awareness Week Kit: Celebrating our natural sizes.National Eating Disorder Information Centre, Toronto, Canada.

4. Kaplan A, P Garfinkel. Medical issues and eating disorders. 1993. Brunner/Mazel,NY.

5. Alexander-Mott. *See 1.*

6. Alexander-Mott. *See 1.*

7. Berg F. Eating disorders — physical and mental effects. Healthy Weight J., Mar/Apr 1995;9:2:27-30.

8. Levine M. Prevalence of eating disorders, some tentative facts, for EDAP, Feb 1 1996.

9. Sesan R. Feminist inpatient treatment for eating disorders. Fallon, *see Ch2:2:251.*

10. Hoek H. The distribution of eating disorders. In Eating Disorders and Obesity, edit K Brownell and C Fairburn. Guilford Press, NY. 1995:207-211.

11. Position of the American Dietetic Association: Nutrition intervention in the treatment of anorexia nervosa, bulimia nervosa, and

binge eating. ADA, Chicago.

12. Wilson, GT. The controversy over dieting. Guilford Press, NY 1995:87-92.

13. Reiff, *see Ch3:3,* p312.

14. Allis Tim, et al. Weight and See. People 1/31/94; p 50-58.

15. Berning J, S Steen. Sports Nutr for the 90s. 1991:156-158. Aspen, Gaithesburg, MD.

16. Diagnostic criteria for eating disorders. Diagnostic and Statistical Manual, Fourth Edition, 1994. American Psychiatric Association, Washington, DC.

17. ADA, *See 11.*

18. Krasnow M. My Life as a Male Anorexic. 1996. Haworth Press, N.Y.

19. Are (Were) You like me? The Healthy Weigh 1995;1:1:3.

20. Reiff, *see Ch3:3.*

21. Keys, *see Ch3:4.*

22. Reiff, *see Ch3:3:245.*

23. Berg F. Eating disorders affect mind and body. Healthy Weight J., Mar/Apr 1995; 9:2:27-30. HRWL, *see Ch 2:9:57-58.*

24. Berg F. Competitive bodybuilding. Healthy Weight J., May/Jun 1996;10:3:47-48.

25. Wooley S. Recognition of Sexual Abuse: Progress and Backlash. Schwartz M, L Cohn, editors. Sexual abuse and eating disorders. 1996. Brunner/Mazel, New York.

26. Brewerton T. Sexual and physical assault are risk factors for bulimia nervosa. NEDO Newsletter 1994;7:4:1-5.

27. Schwartz M, L Cohn, eds. Sexual abuse and eating disorders. 1996. Brunner/Mazel,NY.

28. Levenkron S, One man's experience treating a woman's disorder. Renfrew Perspective 1995;1:2:1-15.

29. Fallon, *see Ch2:2.*

30. Kaplan, *see 4.*

Chapter 5

1. Nutrition News 1988;51:2:5-7.
   Berg F. Weight-loss programs for children and adolescents, Criteria for evaluating clinical programs. HWJ/Obesity & Health Mar 1989;3:10:78.

2. Eating and Its Disorders, edit Albert J. Stunkard and Eliot Stellar, 1984, Raven Press, NY. p 175.

3. Dietz, William, and Nevin Scrimshaw. Potential advantages and disadvantages of human obesity, from Social Aspects and Beach Publ. Luxembourg.

4. Brownell Kelly, C Fairburn, Edits. Eating Disorders and Obesity. 1995. Guilford Press, N.Y. p 417-421.

5. Stunkard A, Wadden T. Psychopathology and obesity. Human Obesity, Eds. Wurtman T, J. NY Academy of Sci 1987:57.

6. Report on Size Discrimination, NEA, Adopted Oct. 7, 1994. For more information, contact: Mary Faber, NEA, 1201 16th St., NW, Washington, DC 20036-3290 (202-822-7700; Fax 202-822-7578.

7. Johnson C A, Self-Esteem Comes in All Sizes. 1995:8-10, Doubleday, N.Y.

8. Erdman, C K. Nothing to Lose: A Guide to Sane Living in a Larger Body. 1995. HarperCollins, N.Y.

9. Davis D. Radiance, Fall 1987, p29-31.

10. Mayer K. Real Women don't Diet. 1993:115-116. Bartleby Press, Silver Spring, MD.

11. Brownell, *see 4.*

12. Hall L. Full Lives: Women who have freed themselves from food & weight obsession. 1993. Gurze Books, Carlsbad, CA.

13. Fort Lauderdale Sun-Sentinel August 27, 1996; Canada Wyde, Fall 1996:6. AP Ft. Lauderdale, March 23, 1997.

14. Goodman C. The Invisible Woman: Confronting Weight Prejudice in America. 1995:ix-xi. Gurze Books, Carlsbad, Calif.

15. Summer, N. Teaching kids about size awareness. Healthy Weight Journal 1996;10:5:95-96.

Chapter 6

1. Kumanyika S. Epidemiologic Reviews 1987;9:31-50.

2. Troiano R, K Flegal, et al. Overweight prevalence and trends for children and adolescents. Arch Pediatr Adolesc Med. 1995;149:1085-1091.

3. Berg F. Heaviest children log increases. Healthy Weight J 1997;11:1:6. Obesity Res 1996;4:1S:68S.

4. Shear C, D Freedman, et al. The Bogalusa Heart Study. Am J Public Health 1988;78:75-77.

5. Morrison J, et al. Mothers in black and white households: the NHLBI growth and health study. An J Pub Health 1994;84:1761-1767.
   Obarzanek E, G Schreiber, P Crawford, et al. Energy intake and physical activity in relation to indexes of body fat: the National Heart, Lung, and Blood Institute.

6. Pediatric Nutrition Surveillance System (PedNSS), Division of Nutrition, Centers for Disease Control in Atlanta.
   Berg F. High rates of childhood obesity seen in assistance programs; Overweight hits 10-year high. HWJ/Obesity & health Mar/Apr 1992;6:2:26-27, 34.

7. Berg F. Prevalences of obesity rises for minorities. HWJ/Obesity & Health Jul/Aug 1993;7:4:72.

8. Fontvieille, A M and E Ravussin. Metabolic

Rate and body composition Indian and Caucasian children, Critical Rev in Food Sci and Nutr 1993;33(4/5):363-368.

9. Becque MD, K Hattori, et. al. Em J Phys Anthro 71;423-249.

Berg F. Health Risks of Obesity. 1993. Healthy Weight Journal, ND.

10. Bouchard C, F Johnston. Fat distribution during growth and later health outcomes. 1988. Alan Liss, NY.

Berg, HRO, see 9:43.

Berg F. Ethnic differences in fat patterning. HWJ/International Obesity Newsletter Dec 1988;2:12:5.

11. Lohman T, S Gonig, et al. Concept of chemical immaturity in body composition estiamtes. Am J Hum Biol 1989;1:201-204.

Berg. Definition. HRO, see 9:110.

12. Arch Pediatr Adolesc Med 1995;149

13. Bouchard C, L Perusse, et al. Inheritance of the amount and distribution of human body fat. Int J Obesity 1988;12:205-215

Berg F. NAASO highlights. HWJ/Obesity & Health 1992:6:1:5.

14. Mayer J. Genetic factors in human obesity. Ann NY Acad Sci 1965;131:412-421, Mayer 1965, PubEd wkshop report, p27.

15. Kumanyika S. Epidemiologic Reviews 1987;9:31-50.

Wendorf M, I Goldfine, Diabetes 1991;40:161-165.

Berg F. Thrifty gene may set stage for obesity in blacks, HWJ/Obesity & Health Jan/Feb 1991:5:1:6-7.

Berg F. Former big game hunters succumb to diabetes, HWJ/Obesity & Health Nov/Dec 1991;5:6:98.

Berg F. Thrifty gene threatens the good life, Healthy Weight J., Jul/Aug 1995;9:4:64.

16. Obarzanek, see 5.

17. Obarzanek, see 5.

18. Klesges Robert, J Applied Behavior Analysis, Winter 1983.

HWJ/International Obesity Newsletter Jan 1987.

19. Johnson S, L Birch. Parents' and children's adiposity and eating style. Pediatrics 1994;94:653-661.

20. J Am Diet A 1991 Sp191:9:A-81.

Berg F. Family communication. HWJ/Obesity & Health Mar/Apr 1992;6:2:24.

Berg F. Infants and young children, family tendencies hold strong influence. HWJ/Obesity & Health Dec 1989;3:12:89, 91-92.

21. Mogan J, Int J Nurs Stud 1986;23:3:255-264.

22. Crawford P, L Shapiro. How obesity develops: A new look at nature and nurture.

HWJ/Obesity & Health 1991;5:3:40-41.

Berg F. Fat cells: An increase in number or in size? HWJ/Obesity & health Aug 1988;2:8:1-2.

23. Giblin W P. JADA 1984;436-438.

24. Filer L J. Summary of the Workshop on Child and Adolescent Obesity, University of Critical Reviews in food Science and Nutrition 1993:33:4/5:287-305.

25. Filer. See 23.

26. Epidemiologic Reviews 1987;9:31-50.

Berg, see 15.

27. NIH Strategy Development Workshop for Public Education on Weight and Obesity, sponsored by the National Heart, Lung and Blood Institutes in 1992, p51.

28. Tufts U Diet & Nutr Ltr Jan 1993;1-2.

Berg F. Teen obesity increases heart risk. HWJ/Obesity & Health Mar/Apr 1993;7:2:31.

29. Smoak C, G Burke, et al. Relation of obesity to clustering of risk factors in children. A J of Epidemiology 1987;125:3:364-372.

Berg, HRWL, see 9:24.

30. Berg F. Obesity in children and teens. HWJ/International Obesity Newsl., 1986;pilot:8:1-2.

31. Frisch R, Edit. Adipose Tissue and Reproduction, 1990, Karger, Basel, Switzerland.

Berg F. High body fat brings early puberty. HWJ/Obesity & Health 1990;4:10:73-76.

Berg, HRWL, see Ch2:9:54.

32. Critical Review Food Sci and Nutr 1993;93(4/5);423-430.

33. NIH, PubEd, see 27, p35.

34. Conference on the Prevention of Obesity. NIDDK, 1993:64. Abstracts:64.

Chapter 7

1. Third Report on Nutrition Monitoring, see Ch1:3. Advance Data, MMWR, Nov 14, 1994.

2. Nicklas T. Dietary studies of children: The Bogalusa Heart Study. JADA 1995;95:1127-1133.

3. 7th European Congress on Obesity, Barcelona, Spain. I J Obesity 1996;20(4):53.

4. What and where our children eat: 1994 Nationwide Survey results. USDA News release, Apr 18, 1996.

5. Eaton S B, M Konner. Paleoplithic. NEJM 1985;312:5:283-289.

6. Surgeon General's report on Nutrition and Health, 1988, HHS, PHS.

7. Kretchmer N, J Beard, S Carlson. The role of nutrition in the development of normal cognition. Am J Clin Nutr 1996;63:997S-1001S.

8. Levine P. Connections in primary prevention. The Renfrew Perspective Fall 1995;1:3:5-6.

9. Jarvis W. Why I am not a vegetarian. Nutrition & Health Forum, 1996;13:6:57-64.

10. AMA Statement, Sept 29, 1992.

11. Woolsey M. The eating disordered vegetarian. Healthy Weight J., 1997;11:2:32-34.

12. Pollitt E. Does breakfast make a difference in school? JADA 1995;95:10:1134-1139.

13. Nicklas, *see 2.*

14. Whelan E. Smoking report. Priorities 1996;8:1:4-9.

15. AP Atlanta, Feb. 7, 1997.

16. Sallis, J F. Epidemiology of physical activity and fitness in children and adolescents, Crit Rev in Food Sci and Nutr 1993;33(4/5):403-408.

17. Iverson, et al, Public Health Reports, 1985;100(2):212.

18. The physically underdeveloped child, 1984: 0-438-699. USHHS, President's Council on Physical Fitness, Washington, DC.

19. Iverson. *See 17.*

20. Melpomene J Fall 1993;14-18, 19-26.
Berg F. Why teenage girls drop out of sports. HWJ/Obesity & Health Jan/Feb 1994;8:1:13.

21. Melpomene J Fall 1993;14-18, 19-26.
Berg F. Picture books portray mostly males in sports. HWJ/Obesity & Health 1994;8:1:13.

Chapter 8

1. Dieting and purging behavior in black and white high school students. JADA 1992;92:3:306-312.
Adolescents dieting. JAMA 1991;266:2811-2812.
Berg F. Harmful weight loss practices are widespread among adolescents. HWJ/Obesity & Health Jul/Aug 1992:6:4:69-72.

2. YRBS, *see Ch1:4.*

3. JADA, JAMA, Berg, *see 1.*

4. JADA, JAMA, Berg, *see 1.*

5. JADA, JAMA, Berg, *see 1.*

6. Berg, *see Ch 2:9:50-55.*

7. Garner D, L Rosen. Eating disorders among athletes. J Applied Sport Sci Research 1991;5:2:17.

8. Obesity Research 1993;1:1:51-56.
Berg F. Linking gallstones with weight loss. HWJ/Obesity & Health May/Jun 1993;7:3:45.

9. Options, *see Ch1:12.*

10. JADA, JAMA, Berg, *see 1.*

11. JADA, JAMA, Berg, *see 1.*

12. Kaplan, *see Ch4:4, p101-122.*

13. Clin Psych Rev 1991;11:729-780.

Berg F. Nondiet movement gains strength. HWJ/Obesity & Health Sep/Oct 1992;6:5:85-90.

14. Satter, *see Ch3:11.*

15. Smolak, *see Ch2:19.*

16. Reiff, *see Ch3:3, p162.*

17. Eating Disorder Awareness Week Kit: Celebrating our natural sizes. 1996, National Eating Disorder Information Centre, Toronto.

18. Young M Evans. Diet Breaking: Having it all without having to diet. Hodder and Soughton, London. 1995;41-42, 56-57.

19. Levitsky D. Diet drugs gain popularity. Healthy Weight J., 1997;11:1:8-12.
Ernsberger P. Adverse reactions to dexfenfluramine. Healthy Weight J., 1997;11:1:13-14, 16.

20. Levitsky, Ernsberger, *see 19.*

21. Long-term pharmacotherapy in the management of obesity, National Task Force on the Prevention and Treatment of Obesity. JAMA 1996;276:1907-1915.
Berg F. Task Force advises against diet drugs, Healthy Weight J., 1997;11:2:27.

22. Berg F. The case against PPA. HWJ/Obesity & Health 1991;5:1:9-12.

23. JAMA, JADA, Berg, *see 1.*

24. Kaplan A, P Garfinkel. Medical issues and the Eating Disorders. 1993. Brunner/Mazel, New York.

25. Berg F. 1997 Slim Chance Awards. Healthy Weight J., 1997;11:1:7.

26. Berg F. Weight Loss Quackery and Fads, 1995:16. Healthy Weight J.,, Hettinger, ND.

27. FDA Consumer, May 1995;3.

28. Berg F. Bee pollen "cures" truckers of obesity, tumors, radiation. HWJ/Obesity & Health Mar/Apr 1991;5:2:30.

29. Rosencrans K. Diet pills suspected in deaths. Healthy Weight J., Jul/Aug 1994;8:4:68.

30. Berg, WLQF, *see 26.*

31. Mayer, *see Ch5:10, p149.*

32. Hall, *see Ch5:12, p96-97.*

33. JADA, JAMA, Berg, *see 1.*

34. YRBS, *see Ch1:4.*

35. Baker D and A, R Sansone. Overview of eating disorders. 1994. NEDO.
Berg, *see Ch2:9:40.*

36. Mehler P, K Weiner. Frequently asked medical questions about eating disorder patients. Eating Disorders, 1994;2:1:22-30.

37. Kaplan, *see Ch4:4.*

38. YRBS, *see Ch1:4.*

39. NEJM 1995;333:1165-1170, 1214-1216.
Berg F. Smoking cessation impacts weight. Healthy Weight J., Mar/Apr 1996;10:2:27-28.

40.Healthy People 2000 1990:140, 147. USDHHS, PHS.

41. Williamson D, R Anda, G Giovino, T Byers, CDC, J Madans, Kleinman. Weight gain caused by cessation of smoking. Natl Ctr for Health Statistics. 1993;324:739-745. NEJM, *see 40.*

Berg F. Smokers who quit gain to average. HWJ/Obesity & Health Nov/Dec 1991;5:6:92.

42. Rand C, A MacGregor. Adolescents having obesity surgery. Southern Med J, 1994;87:12:1208-1213.

43. Bloomers T, Exec Mgr Am Society for Bariatric Surgery, interview 1994;5.

44. Guidance for Treatment of Adult Obesity, 1996. Shape Up America! and American Obesity Assoc.

45. Questionable feature, each issue. Slim Chance Awards, each Jan. Healthy Weight Journal. See also Weight Loss Quackery and Fads, 1995. HWJ.

46. Kratina K. Exercise dependence. 1995. Eds: K King Helm, B Klawitte. Nutrition Therapy: Advanced counseling skills. In press.

47. Berg, HRWL, *see Ch 2:9:24-38.*

48. Garner, *see 7:100-107.*

Berg, HRWL, *see Ch 2:9:55.*

49. Steen S, S McKinney. Nutrition assessment of college wrestlers. Phys Sportsmed 1986;14:100-116.

Berg F. Weight cycling; crash dieting drops metabolism for wrestlers; Wrestling with weight. HWJ/Obesity & Health Feb 1989;3:2:1-4.

Berg, HRWL, *see Ch2:9:52.*

50. Wisconsin Interscholastic Athletic Association, 41 Park Ridge Drive, PO Box 267, Stevens Point, WI 54481; 715Ä344Ä8580.

51. Muscle & Fitness. Feb 1996:137-138, 221-222.

52. Dwyer E, D Silbiger, J Ryan. The red flags of over-training. Shape Apr 1996;122-123.

53. Dwyer, *see 52.*

54. Food & Nutr News Nov/Dec 1989;61:5

Berg F. Summer weight loss camps: Not a quick fix for overweight teens. HWJ/Obesity & Health Mar 1990;4:3:29.

55. AP Feb 27, 1991.

56. Guidance, *see 44.*

57. Fraser L. Losing it: America's obsession with weight and the industry that feeds on it. 1997. Dutton, Penquin, N.Y.

58. Berg F. The weight loss industry. Regulation is needed. HWJ/Obesity & Health Jun 1990;4:6:41-46.

59. NIH Technology Conf., *see Ch1:14.* Also: Annals Int Med 1993;119:688-770.

60. Berg, *see 58.*

61. NIH. *See Ch 1:14.*

Chapter 9

1. Miller W. Health promotion strategies for obese patients. Healthy Weight J., 1997:11:3:47-51.

Barlow et al. Int J Obesity 1995;19:S41-S44.

2. Options, *see Ch 1:12.*

3. Satter E. The new paradigm of trust. Healthy Weight J., Nov/Dec 1995;9:6:107-108. Satter, *see Ch 3:11.*

4. Berg F. Nutritionists call for new approach. HWJ/Obesity & Health May/Jun 1991;5:3:36.

Ikeda J. If My Child is Too Fat, What Should I do About it? Nutrition Education, Cooperative Extension, Dept. of Nutritional Sciences, University of California, Berkeley.

5. Vitality, *see Ch 1:5.*

6. Search Institute, Healthy communities, healthy youth. 7000 S 3rd St, #210, Minneapolis, MN 55415 (1-800-888-7828, Fax 612-376-8956, http://www.search-institute.org)

Chapter 10

1. Search, Healthy communities, *see Ch 9:6.*

2. Satter *see Ch 3:11.*

3. Hans, C, RD, D Nelson. A parent's guide to children's weight. 1994. Iowa State Extension Service, Iowa State U, Ames, 50011.

4. Walsh K. Nutrition for busy families I. Herald-Press Mar 8, 1997, Fessenden, N.D.

5. Fortin S, Supporting adolescents with eating problems: Suggestions for the family. National Eating Disorder Information Centre Bulletin. 1995;10:2:1-4.

6. Johnson S, L Birch. Parents' adiposity and childrens's adiposity and eating style. Pediatrics 1994;94:653-660.

7. Crawford P, MPH RD, L Shapior, DrPH, RD. How obesity develops: a new look at nature and nurture. HWJ/Obesity & Health May/Jun 1991;5:3:40-41.

8. I J Eat Disorders 1986;5:335-346.

9. Satter E, MS, MSSW, RD. Childhood obesity demands new approaches. HWJ/Obesity & Health 1991;5:3:42-43. 5.

Satter E. Internal regulation and the evolution of normal growth as the basis for prevention of obesity in childhood. J Am Diet Assoc. In press.

Diag/Stat Manual IIIR, 1988. Am Psych Assoc

10. Bruch. Eating Disorders. Basic Books, 1973.

11. Satter, see *Ch 9:3, see also 9.*

12. Ikeda J, et al. Two approaches to adolescent weight reduction. J Nutr Educ 1982;14:90.

13. Ikeda J. Winning weight loss for teens. 1989. Bull Publishing, Palo Alto, CA.
14. Ikeda J, MA, RD, E Peck, DPH, RD. California takes action on children weight concerns. HWJ/Obesity & Health 1991;5:3:39.
15. Ikeda, *see Ch 9:4.*
16. Johnson C, MA. 1995. Reprinted with permission from materials compiled by Largely Positive, Inc. Glendale, Wisc.
17. Johnson, *see Ch 5:7.*

Chapter 11

1. Allensworth D, L Kolbe. Comprehensive school health program. J School Hlth1987 57;10:409-412.
2. Kolbe L. An essential strategy to improve the health and education of Americans. 55-80. From Cortese P, K Middleton edits. The Comprehensive School Health Challenge, Vol 1: Promoting health through education. 1994. ETR Assoc., Santa Cruz, CA.
3. National Assoc. to Advance Fat Acceptance. 225 30th St., Sacramento, CA, 95816.
4. Summer, *see Ch5:15.*
5. Piran N. On prevention and transformation. The Renfrew Perspective. 1996;2:1:8-9.
6. Estes L, M Crago, C Shisslak. Eating Disorders Prevention. The Renfrew Perspective. 1996;2:1:3-5.
7. Smolak, Levine, *see Ch2:19.*
8. Levine P, see *Ch2:28.*
9. Eating Disorders Awareness and Prevention (EDAP), 603 Stewart Street #803, Seattle, WA 98101 (206-382-3587; fax 206-292-9890) http://members.aol.com/edapinc.
10. NIH Strategy Workshop*, see Ch6:27.*
11. Omichinski L. Teens & Diets: No Weigh. HUGS International, Portage la Prairie, Manitoba, Canada.
12. Food & Nutrition News Mar/Apr 1995:67:2:1-4.
13. Johnston J, P Marmet, et al. Kansas LEAN: an effective coalition for nutrition education and dietary change. J Nutr Ed 1996;28:2:115-118.
14. Sallis J. Strategy Development Workshop for Public Education on Weight, NHLBI, Sept. 1992.
15. Project SPARK, Sports Play and Active Recreation for Kids, research project funded by National Heart, Lung and Blood Institute, March 1995. For more information: Judy Folkenberg, NIH Healthline, Bldg 31, Rm 2B10, Bethesda, MD 20892, 301-496-1766.

16. Wisconsin, *see Ch8:50.*

Chapter 12

1. Vitality, *see Ch 1:5.*
2. Beck P. Vegetarian Diets. Aug 1990. NDSU Extension Service, Fargo, N.D.
3. Olson R. Folly of restricting fat in the diet of children. Nutrition Today 1995;30:6:234-245.
4. Reiner S. CLA: Does fat have a silver lining? Priorities 1996;3:4:42-47.
5. Reaching consumers with meaningful health messages: Putting the Dietary Guidelines into action. 1996. Dietary Guidelines Alliance.
6. Hans, *see Ch10:3.*
7. Johnston G. New vision for exercise. HWJ/Obesity & Health Nov/Dec 1992;6:6:108.
8. Sallis, *see Ch7:16; Ch11:13, 14.* Sallis, *see Ch 11:15.*
9. Jaffee L, P Wu. After-school activities and self-esteem in adolescent girls. Melpomene J, summer 1996;15:2:18-25; Shape Nov. 1995.
10. JADA 1995;95:1414-1417. Berg F. Avoid weight loss focus. Healthy Weight J., 1996;10:4:75.
11. Melpomene J Fall 1993; 14-26. Berg F. Why teenage girls drop out of sports. HWJ/Obesity & Health Jan/Feb 1994;8:1:13.

Chapter 13

1. Healthy Weight Week awards. Healthy Weight J., 1997:11:1:5.
2. Pipher, *see Ch2:1.*
3. Huon G. Health promotion and the prevention of dieting-induced disorders. Eat Disorders 1996;4:1:27-32.
4. NEA, *see Ch5:6.*
5. Larkin, *see Ch2:30.*
6. Whelan E. Priorities 1996;8:1:4-9.

Chapter 14

1. Berg, HRWL, *see Ch 2:9.*
2. Berg F. Connecticut law curbs diet claims. Healthy Weight Journal 1996;10:6:109. Law effective Oct.1, 1996 (SHB 5621;Pub Act 96-126). For information contact: Conn. Dept Consumer Protection, 165 Capitol Ave., Hartford CT 06106 (203-566-4499; fax 203-566-7630).
3. Am J Clin Nutr 1994;60:153-156. Berg F. Is drug abuse the next miracle cure? Healthy Weight J., Sep/Oct 1994;8:5:84.

Chart references

Chapter 3

1. Berg F. Dysfunctional eating: A new concept. Healthy Weight Journal 1996;10:5:88-92.
2. Garner and Garfinkel's Eating Attitudes Test, Children's version, by Maloney et. al. J Am Academy Chi Adol Psychiatry 1988;27:542-54.
   Allison D. Handbook of Assessment Methods for Eating Behaviors and Weight-Related Problems 1995;488-489. Sage Publ. Thousand Oaks, CA.

Chapter 4

1. Diagnostic criteria for eating disorders. Diagnostic and Statistical Manual, Fourth Edit. 1994. American Psychiatric Assoc., Washington, DC.
2. NEDO materials. National Eating Disorders Organization, 6655 S Yale Ave, Tulsa, OK 74136.

Chapter 6

1. Troiano R, et al. Overweight prevalence and trends for children and adolescents. Arch Pediat Adolesc Med 1995;149:1085-1091.
2. Update: Prevalence of overweight among children, adolescents and adults — U.S., 1988-1994. MMWR March 7, 1997;46:9:199-202. See also 1.
3. See 2.
4. Bouchard C, F Johnston. Fat distribution during growth and later health outcomes. 1988. Alan Liss, New York.
   Berg F. Ethnic differences in fat patterning. HWJ/Obesity & Health Dec 1988;2:12:5.
   Berg F. Health Risks of Obesity. 1995;43. Healthy Weight J., Hettinger, ND.
5. Klesges R. J Applied Behavior Analysis. Winter 1983.

Chapter 7

1. National Center for Health Statistics. Unpublished data, 1997. NHANES III, Phase 1, 1988-91.
2. NCHS, see 1.
3. NCHS, see 1.
4. Youth Risk Behavior Surveillance - US, 1995. Morbidity and Mortality Weekly Report, CDC, US Public Health Service. Sept 27, 1996;45:SS-4.
5. 1995 NHIS-YRBS surveys. See 4. Surgeon General's Report on Physical Activity and Health, NHIS-YRBS data, 1996, CDC, HHS, PHS.

Chapter 8

1. Dieting and purging behavior in black and white high school students. JADA 1992;92:3:306-312.
   Berg F. Harmful weight loss practices are widespread among adolescents. HWJ/Obesity & Health Jul/Aug 1992;6:4:69-72.
2. Berg F. Health Risks of Weight Loss, 1995. Healthy Weight Journal, Hettinger, ND.
3. YRBS, see Ch 7:4.
4. King A. A doctor's weight loss education. HWJ/Obesity & Health guest editorial Nov/Dec 1993;7:6:104.

Chapter 9

1. Vitality Leader's Kit. 1994. Health Services and Promotion, Health and Welfare Canada, Ottawa.

Chapter 10

1. Wisconsin Dept. of Health and Social Services.
2. Smolak L, PhD, M Levine, PhD. Ten things parents can do to help prevent eating disorders in their children. NEDO Newsletter, Summer 1994;3. Healthy Weight J., Sep/Oct 1995;9:5:92.
   Levine M P, PhD. Ten things Men Can Do and Be to Help Prevent Eating Disorders. NEDO Newsletter, Apr/May 1994. Healthy Weight Journal Jan/Feb 1995;9:1:15. National Eating Disorders Org., 445 E Granville Rd, Worthington, OH 43085.
3. Chaussee S, LSW. Eating disorders prevention, 1992. Archway Family Services, PO Box 5510, St. Alexius Medical Center Bismarck, ND, 58502.
4. NEDO, see 2.
5. Ikeda J. With permission, from If My Child Is Too Fat, What Should I Do About It? Booklet for parents. University of Calif.
6. Satter E. Feeding with Love and Good Sense: Training Manual. 1995. Ellyn Satter Associates, 4226 Mandan Crescent, Madison, WI 53711.

Chapter 12

1. Dietary Guidelines for Americans. 1995. USDA, USDHHS.
2. Healthy People 2000. Midcourse Revisions. 1994. USDHHS, Public Health Service.

Index

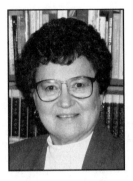

A licensed nutritionist and family wellness specialist, **FRANCES M. BERG, M.S., LN**, is the editor, founder and publisher of *Healthy Weight Journal* and an internationally known authority on weight and eating issues. Berg's weekly health column, *Healthy Living,* has been published in over 50 newspapers. An Adjunct Professor at the University of North Dakota School of Medicine, she is the author of eight books, and has presented at numerous national conferences. Her master's degree in family social science and anthropology is from the University of Minnesota, and she holds a Home Economics (Family and Consumer Science) degree from Montana State University.

Berg serves on the Boards of Directors of the American Diabetes Association, N.D. affiliate, and the West River Regional Medical Center. She is National Coordinator of the Task Force on Weight Loss Abuse for the National Council Against Health Fraud, and a member of the Society for Nutrition Education, Academy for Eating Disorders, North American Association for the Study of Obesity, the National Association to Advance Fat Acceptance, and the Society for the Study of Ingestive Behavior. She has four children and lives with her husband in Hettinger, North Dakota.

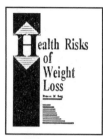
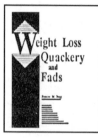
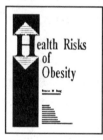
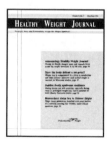

America's children are afraid to eat!

It's a fear that consumes them, shatters lives, even kills.

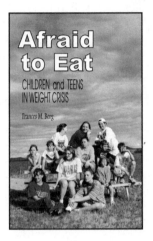

At last! A book that challenges America's obsession with weight and the lengths to which this drives young people. *Afraid to Eat* explains how this is harming kids and shows the way to healthful change.

Learn about these issues:
- Why teenage girls "hate" their bodies
- How eating disorders destroy lives
- Why one in five teenagers is overweight
- How daily humiliation punishes large kids
- And the challenge of promoting wellness and wholeness for every child of every size!

ORDER NOW to get the facts you need!

✔ **YES! I want to receive the top resource in the field of healthy eating and weight. Please send me immediately _____ copies of** *Afraid to Eat.*

_____ $17.95 softcover   _____ $24.95 hardcover

NAME --

ADDRESS --

                                                                TELEPHONE

Total enclosed $_____
❑ Visa   ❑ MasterCard

Card # _ _ _ _ _ _ _ _ _ _ _ _ _ _ _ _

Exp. date_____

Signature_____

POSTAGE: U.S.–$3.00 1st book, $1 each additional; Foreign–$3.00 surface each; $9.00 airmail.

Guarantee: Your satisfaction 100% guaranteed or receive a full refund, no questions asked.

HEALTHY WEIGHT PUBLISHING NETWORK
402 SOUTH 14TH STREET, HETTINGER, ND 58639 ● www.HealthyWeightNetwork.com

"A MUCH NEEDED BOOK . . . The reader is immediately impressed by the book's cover — not perfectly poised or air-brushed bodies, but rather "real" kids, all sizes and shapes, all different thoughts and feelings, all unique individuals . . .

"Berg dares to speak out on behalf of parents, educators, health professionals, and all members of society. She believes that different groups are working at cross-purposes despite their best intentions.

"The news (on nutrient deficiencies) should be alarming, but the media's attention is fixated on obesity fear rather than the long-term health problems associated with growth and development. Chapter 3 nicely develops the concept of dysfunctional eating, one of the most underreported and least publicized eating patterns among our youth today. . .

"Berg skillfully uses personal accounts to depict the horrific pain that large children and teens endure. This is an issue that should touch our hearts deeply, make us angry, and give us motivation to bring about change in our school system. Inspires the reader to action.

— *EATING DISORDERS: Journal of Treatment & Prevention*

"AFRAID TO EAT is the first attempt to present the devastating effects of our culture's obsession with thinness and dieting on all of our children. It should serve as a call to action for all parents, educators and health care professionals in America."

— *Joseph McVoy, PhD*
Director, Association for the Health Enrichment of Large People

"THERE'S A SILENT EPIDEMIC so large and extreme, it could only happen in this weight-obsessed culture: children's fear of eating. Six-year-olds understand that fat is undesirable and by fourth grade, 40 percent or more of girls "diet" at least occasionally. A survey of young girls revealed that they were more afraid of becoming fat than they were of cancer, nuclear war or losing their parents. That is some of the bad news.

"The good news is that *Healthy Weight Journal* editor Berg, is out to change these attitudes. This is the most important book on eating problems of the young. Berg's solution is a benign health promotion approach that focuses on good health for all children, recognizes the connection between eating and weight problems, and seeks to strengthen the positive aspects of culture, family and friends.

"Her call to action is loud, clear, and above all, provides the framework for change. Anyone involved in shaping the eating habits of the young must read this book, especially parents and teachers."

— *CHOICE, American Library Association*

"**A SUPERB JOB** of pulling together the facts and research! *Afraid to Eat* equips educators to work with teens with confidence. Provides examples of what to expect when working with this group, i.e. teens use vegetarianism as a way to diet, and camouflage it as healthy eating. Thoughtful insight . . . detailed references."

— *Linda Omichinski, RD*
President, HUGS International

"*AFRAID TO EAT* **EXTENSIVELY DOCUMENTS** the tragic results of our society's preoccupation with achievement of the ideal body, particularly the impact it has on children and adolescents.

"The author points out how the medical profession's insistence on achievement of ideal weight as a national health priority has reinforced and validated this obsession with body size and shape. Instead of resulting in improved health, efforts that were supposed to help people manage their weight, have backfired, contributing to an epidemic of body dissatisfaction, size discrimination, restrictive eating, bizarre eating disorders, poor nutrition, and increased depression, anxiety, frustration, and low self-esteem among our nation's youth.

"Fortunately, Berg does not stop there. The second half of her book is devoted to how we can rectify this situation and nurture our youth in positive ways that enhance their physical, emotional, and social well-being. She suggests that we abandon our weight centered approach to health promotion and embrace a paradigm that emphasizes self-empowerment, body trust, and self acceptance. Berg's book makes a significant contribution toward documenting and suggesting how we can handle a major crisis that has been too long ignored."

— *Joanne Ikeda, MA, RD*
California Extension Nutrition Education Specialist
NAAFA Newsletter